THE
OMEGA
CONNECTION

THE
OMEGA
CONNECTION

The facts about fish oils and human health

S. K. Niazi, Ph.D.
Health Sciences Center
University of Illinois at Chicago
Chicago, Illinois

Esquire Books, Inc.

Nothing contained herein is to be construed as a diet recommended or endorsed by the author or the publisher. Individuals should not attempt to diagnose, treat or use measures to prevent diseases without consulting a physician.

Figures 2.2, 5.1 and 5.2 after DeBakey, M., et al. *The Living Heart Diet.* Raven 1984.

Library of Congress Cataloging-in-Publication Data

Niazi, S. K. (Sarfaraz Khan), 1949-
    The Omega Connection.
    Bibliography; p.
    Includes Index.
    1. Omega-3 fatty acids--Therapeutic use
    2. Omega-3 fatty acids--physiological effect.
    3. Fish oils in human nutrition. I. Title.
[DNLM: 1. Fatty acids, Unsaturated--popular
works 2. Fish oils--popular works. 3. Fishes--
popular works. QU 90 N557o]
RM 666.O45N53 1987   615'.34   86-82991
ISBN 0-9617841-0-5
87 88 88 89 90   5 4 3 2 1

To Omayr, Ali and Nabiha
whose tiffs are as comforting to the heart
as omega-3 fatty acids.

WITHDRAWN

"No human being, however great, or powerful, was ever so free as a fish."

JOHN RUSKIN, The Two Paths. Lecture 5.

CONTENTS

Page

JAN 1990

LIST OF TABLES, FIGURES AND APPENDICES

TABLE Page

FIGURE

APPENDIX

ACKNOWLEDGEMENTS

Thanks are due to my colleagues at the University of Illinois and the hundreds of dedicated researchers, whose findings make this book. I am especially indebted to the stimulating discussions with Dr. Frederick Siegel, Dr. Alvin Shemesh, Mr. Jamil Rahman, Mr. Donald Pipping, and Mr. David Ghezzi. The writings of Dr. William E. M. Lands, a renowned expert on how fish affects human health, have greatly inspired me. I have also benefitted immensely from the editorial comments of Ms. Virginia Mullery.

PREFACE

The fault may not lie in your stars, but in your diet. More people die in this country due to diseases inflicted by food than from all other reasons combined. But don't despair. Science has just discovered how to make food healthy and enjoyable again. This is not just additional advice on sensible eating, instead, it is about eating what makes most sense. You are what you eat, or so goes an old saying. Wouldn't all of us rather be cool, supple, agile, lean and calm, like a fish? This is a story about FISH, the most potent panacea for all human ailments. The pages of this book unfold the mysteries of the most deadly diseases, the role of diet in causing or exacerbating these diseases and how the preventive actions of fish can change the course of these diseases. It's an intelligent approach, based on scientific findings, to make you believe what you may have already heard from old wives' tales. This book should should serve as a convincing reference and add a few good years to your life.

Dr. S. K. Niazi

1
THE FISH TALE

*"Every man should eat and drink, and
enjoy the good of all his labour, it is
the gift of God."*

Bible, Ecclesiastes 3:13

Americans are living a good life and it's killing them. Despite modern technology and medical advances, they are two to three times more likely to die of cardiovascular diseases and cancer than their forebears at the turn of the century. Three out of four deaths in the U.S. today are related to these two dread diseases.

Despite the fact that the U.S. Congress enacted a law in October 1986, eliminating the mandatory retirement age for Americans, many will not live long enough to reap its benefits.

We spend several hundred billion dollars to take care of our heart and cancer patients per year. Many more billions are wasted in lost productivity and in the expensive replacement of skilled workers.

Heart diseases and cancer are attributes of our lifestyle, environment and eating habits. Unfortunately, we exercise little control over our environment and lifestyle, leaving dietary habits as the major weapon in our fight against these dread diseases. The typical American diet contains too much red meat and fat, too many chemicals and calories, too little fiber, and is often deficient in essential nutrients, vitamins and minerals. This is the result of intense commercialization of the food industry, American life on the fast track and lack of proper education about nutrition. It is ironic that we have successfully conquered the diseases caused by microoranisms but have failed pitifully in containing the diseases caused by the macroorganism, man himself.

Yet in some parts of Russia and northern Pakistan, people commonly live to be 100. They drink, they smoke but they eat simple, high fiber, low fat diets and live considerably tension-free lives. And by so doing, they beat all the odds of Western man against living long.

About 300 miles north of the polar circle lives another race of people who defy all the rules of a healthy diet: they eat raw fat and raw meat for survival. This group of people also beats the odds of dying of heart disease. How? And why? That's a fish tale.

THE INUIT CONNECTION

The Eskimos or Inuits (meaning people who eat raw meat) of northwest Greenland are relatively free of heart disease, diseases of the immune system and have a much lower incidence of many other diseases (table 1.1). In one Eskimo settlement of 1,300 people, the death rate from heart disease was reported to be 3.5 percent as compared to more than 50 percent in most of the Western population. The Eskimos also have almost no asthma, psoriasis, multiple sclerosis or diabetes. This apparent immunity of Eskimos to many diseases had long been attributed to genetics until it was revealed that the Danes, who are of the same Mongolian race as the Eskimos, have more than ten times the risk of dying of heart disease than the Eskimos. However, the Eskimos and the Danes have vastly different eating habits. Although both Eskimos and Danes take about 40 percent of their total calories as fats, the differences in the type of fat used by Danes and Eskimos led researchers to the eventual conclusion that it is the fish and blubber in the Eskimo diet that protects them from heart disease.

TABLE 1.1

INCIDENCE OF DISEASE IN ESKIMOS

Disease	% Difference from Danes
Nonexistent or very low incidence	
Heart attacks	−93
Multiple sclerosis	nonexistent
Psoriasis	−95
Hyperactgive thyroid	nonexistent
Asthma	−96
Diabetes	−90
Low incidence	
Ulcer	−34
Cancer	−14

Higher incidence

Epilepsy	+200
Arterial swelling	+67
Psychosis	+25

The increased incidence of psychoses or nervous disorders in the Eskimos is partly attributed to climactic maladjustments, the increased arterial swelling is probably a side effect of high fat diet (details later) but the reason for higher epileptic seizures in Eskimos can, at best, be only conjectured—a possible effect of eating raw meat?

Similar immunity to diseases has also been recorded in the native Alaskans and populations of fishing villages in Japan. The only common thread between these populations is their diet which is responsible for the health effects observed and not their genes as assumed for many years.

At first glance the Eskimos' diet would seem to be a cardiologist's nightmare. It is very high in animal fat and cholesterol with practically no vegetables, grains or fruit. It consists mainly of raw or cooked seal, whale, fish, caribou and other Arctic wildlife. However, the excess amount of fish in the diet of Eskimos counteracts the deleterious effects of the rest of their diet. The fish contributes a special type of fat called omega-3 fat; the diet of the Western population, on the other hand, is rich in the saturated and unsaturated omega-6 type fats, both of which are now considered harmful to health.

For years, scientists have been searching for reasons why Western man is so predisposed to heart disease and other ailments, but now we have started to look into why others do not die of the same diseases. This turnaround in research emphasis has been extremely useful. Hundreds of researchers from around the world have now put together their findings on the topic and these findings point to only one conclusion: a fish a day can keep the doctor away.

THE DUTCH CONNECTION

In 1965, a group of Dutch scientists visited the town of Zutphen in the Netherlands, where the residents' fish eating habits were diverse. About 20 percent of the population ate no fish while others ate from 1 to 307 gram a day. The Dutch scientists selected about 900 middle aged men who had no history of heart disease for a long-term study of the effects of their dietary habits on heart diseases. Twenty years later, the health histories of these subjects revealed some startling findings (table 1.2). Eating fish made the difference whether the people in Zutphen developed heart disease or not.

TABLE 1.2

FISH DIET AND INCIDENCE OF HEART DISEASE

Fish Consumed (pounds/year)	Incidence
0	average
1-11	40% reduction
12-23	43% reduction
24-35	54% reduction
over 35	58% reduction

Residents of Zutphen who consumed even a small quantity of fish per day had significant protection from heart disease. This study provided an instant credibility to the sporadic observations that fish can be good for the heart.

Similar observations were made in Norway, where it was shown that after World War II, the incidence of heart disease reduced significantly. This was ascribed to dietary changes caused by the German occupation and the consequent food shortage necessitating drastic reduction in dairy fat intake and a substantial increase in fish consumption, which was the only abundant souce of protein and fat available. In Japan, where fish consumption has traditionally been high, low incidence of heart disease is reported.

These discoveries relating heart disease to diet explain why, despite reduced use of saturated fat, the incidence of heart disease has not declined proportionally in many Western countries. The fat Eskimos consume comes from marine sources whereas our foods are rich in fat from animal, vegetable and artificial sources. The differences in the type of fat in our diets determine how fragile our hearts become and how susceptible we remain to other malignancies affecting our body.

OLD WIVES' TALES

Old wives' tales, anecdotes and myths have long touted the beneficial effects of fish. Recent research has given them scientific credence. Discoveries, most of which were concluded in the late 1970s and 1980s, regarding the effect of fish diet, though not unexpected, surprised the medical community in their magnitude and shattered many misconceptions.

For example, some types of fish have long been considered harmful because of their "high" content of saturated fats and cholesterol; the new discoveries show that all types of fish are good for health. Fatty fish such as salmon and shellfish, which were considered equivalent to eggs and lard, are now freely recommended as are oysters, clams and scallops because fish of all types are rich in a type of fat which is good for the heart—omega-3 fat.

Dr. William P. Castelli, Director of the Farmington Heart Study, made a charming statement on reducing risk of heart disease by avoiding saturated fats: "I like to point out to people that if you can't be a vegetarian yourself, eat a vegetarian from the sea." Vegetarians from the sea are oysters, clams and scallops. These dramatic changes in the dietary recommendations have come as a result of many conclusive studies of Eskimos and others who make heavy use of fish as their daily staple.

TABLE 1.3

WHO IS EATING FISH

Population	Pounds/yr/person
Eskimos	325
Okinawans (Japan)	163
Japanese, average	85
Americans	less than 15

Historically, the consumption of fish in the U.S. and many European countries has been lowest in the entire world, despite increases of about 40 percent during the past 35 years (table 1.3). The fish consumption in the U.S. declined slightly in the mid-sixties and has risen slightly since then. Our disinterest in the creatures living in deep water is reflected by our insignificant fish catches compared to our population (table 1.4).

TABLE 1.4

WHO IS CATCHING FISH

Country	% World Catch
Japan	15
USSR	12
USA	5
Peru	5
Norway	4

Westerners in general have not yet developed a "taste" for fish. For many, also, there remains a mystique about the sea, stemming from the old legends of mermaids, Loch Ness monsters and spells of the Bermuda Triangle. And now comes yet another nautical tale which promises to turn our pipe dreams of a long life into a reality.

This book explores the claims, controversies and myths regarding the consumption of fish. We will examine the diseases as well as the cures, the pros as well as the cons, the myths as well as the realities.

2

THE OIL INSIDE YOU

"I think the devil
will not have me damned,
lest the oil that's in me
should set hell on fire."

Shakespeare,
The Merry Wives of Windsor.
Act v, sc. 5, 1. 38.

Some years ago, say a few million, mankind had not yet discovered McNuggets® and Whoppers® and had to make do with whatever catches could be made during good weather. We survived those tough times by developing the ability to store fat as a reserve source of energy. This evolutionary change saved man from extinction. However, with excess storage of fat came many deadly diseases. Fortunately, the process of evolution is a continuous one and now that we do not need such high deposits of fat, help is on the way. Within the next few million years, the human race will not be faced with the dilemma of fighting the battle of bulges as our bodies adjust to the lower fat requirements. In the meantime, however, we must learn to live with our body fats.

Living with our body fats can be made easier, we have recently learned, if we incorporate some fish fat into our diet. Fish fat helps to rearrange, dissolve or otherwise neutralize other fats in the body. How this is done will be examined in this chapter.

WHAT IS FAT?

Fat, as we know it, is a greasy substance which ranges from cooking oil to a beer belly. Americans have a love-hate relationship with fat: they love to take almost 60 percent of their calories as fats but hate being overweight. Almost 80 percent of them are constantly striving to lose weight, most often fruitlessly.

Whatever your reaction to fat, you should realize it is essential to body functions, and in this context, is perhaps more essential than proteins and carbohydrates. The U.S. government classifies fat as an essential nutritional group; however, unlike other nutritional groups, there are no minimum requirements suggested since we always receive enough of it in our diets. Following are some of the important functions of fat in the body:

- **Energy Source:** Fat is the highest source of energy (about 9.5 calories per gram), giving twice as much energy as carbohydrates. The body stores fat as deposits to provide energy on demand. These deposits turn over frequently and are not stagnant tissues, as commonly believed. The carbohydrates and proteins convert to fat before they are utilized as sources of energy. Would you believe, there is no instant energy gained by taking a quick bite of a chocolate bar?

- **Body Insulation:** The fat under our skin and around the vital organs such as the kidneys, liver and womb protects against temperature change and injuries. It was the fat in our body that helped us survive the inclement weather when we used to live in caves and on top of trees. Several species, such as whales, still rely on body fat for survival. Traveling more than 5,000 miles, each way, from Alaska's Bering Sea to warm-water breeding grouds off Baja California, whales rely heavily on their fat deposits for nutrition and protection against weather. (The migration of 12,000 to 13,000 California gray whales each winter is an spectacular event. The two-month, 5,000 mile trek is the longest annual migration by a mammal. January, when the migration hits its peak, is considered the best month for whale-watching—as many as 200 whales a day have been spotted off San Diego's coast line during mid-month. A whale-watching station at Cabrillo National Monument on Point Loma offers free access to a glassed-in observatory as well as to exhibits and a taped presentation about the whales' trek. For information call the Natural History Museum at 619-232-3821.)

Our body resists losing fat because of its essential purpose. Women, who have about 5-10 percent more fat than men, need it specifically during gestational and nursing periods.

• **Chemical Storage:** The fat depcsits in our body often serve as inert reservoirs for many chemicals such as environmental pollutants, carcinogens and drugs to which we are frequently exposed. Without such storage ability, some beneficial drugs would have more dangerous side effects and have to be taken so frequently as to make them useless. Chemicals found in our environment are rendered less dangerous by this chemical storage because they are removed from circulation.

• **Chemical Messengers:** Body functions such as blood clotting, blood pressure, immunity against cancer and infections, inflammation, etc. are all controlled by several chemical messengers synthesized from fats; examples include prostaglandins (PGs), leukotrienes (LTs) and hydroxyeicosatetraenoic acids (HETEs).

Given all these important functions, how can fat

be bad? The answer is an old cliche: too much of a good thing can be bad. Now let's examine how this applies to our body.

HOW LEAN ARE YOU?

Before examining the bad effects of what is around our waist, let's figure out how much of it we carry around. The percentage of body fat is generally calculated by skin fold thickness and body density measurements; but the following simple equation should work for most of us.

$$\text{Percent fat} = [90 - 2(\text{height} - \text{girth})]$$

The girth is measured at just above the umbilical level and the height is without shoes, both expressed in inches. Let us use this equation to calculate the percent of body fat in an 18-year-old who weighs 150 pounds, is 5 ft 2 inches tall and has a waist of 30 inches.

$$\text{Percent body fat} = [90 - 2(62 - 30)] = 26\%$$

The total fat in the body, therefore, is 0.26 x 150 pounds or 39 pounds, which is equivalent to 173,518 calories stored in the body, sufficient for about 115 days at the rate of 1,500 calories per day.

On an average, approximately 15 percent of body weight in men and 25 percent in women is made up of fat, corresponding to about 24 pounds of fat in men and 37 pounds of fat in women. The higher fat in women is necessary to provide for gestational and nursing requirements. In older age, the percent of body fat content increases as the lean muscles wither away.

How much fat we accumulate in our body depends on the number and the size of fat cells. Fat cells form early in life; after adolescence, the formation of new fat cells is quite limited. Therefore, if you were over-weight at an early age, it was due to large number of fat cells, but if you picked up weight after adolescence, it was due mainly to the growth in the size of the existing fat cells. This explains why it is more difficult to rid yourself of childhood obesity.

Adult obesity is more responsive to weight reduc-tion by dietary measure and is much easier to control. The word "easier," however, is a relative one. Those of us who have weight problems know that it is anything but easy to lose weight, despite the plethora of gadgets, gizmos, potions and therapies available to us.

There is no doubt that being overweight causes many diseases, especially heart diseases and cancer, but it is difficult to assess what is the right amount of fat for one person, because of the differences in the metabolism of fat in individuals and how it causes diseases. Most height-weight tables are at best a crude indication of what your weight should be since they do not take into account the high variability in the effect of weight on body functions. The current medical find-ings show that being slightly overweight is more health-ful than being very lean.

As W. S. Gilbert said in "Iolanthe," act I, "I see no objection to stoutness–in moderation."

The havoc fat wreaks on our physical health is,

perhaps, minuscule compared to what it does to our mental health. Only about 8 percent of American elementary-school-age girls are overweight but more than 80 percent of them are on some type of weight-loss program, causing severe nutritional imbalance and leading to such diseases as bolemia, nervosa anorexia and suicidal tendency. The word is out: fat is ugly. Historically, this was not the case. During the Renaissance, for example, pleasingly plump bodies drew great admiration. Food has now become so abundant and cheap due to the technological revolution that eating is no longer only a rich man's indulgence. Consequently, the plump body is no longer in vogue.

INSIDE FAT MOLECULES

The fat in our food is mostly composed of molecules called triglycerides, which are made up of three fatty-acid and one glycerol molecule (figure 2.1).

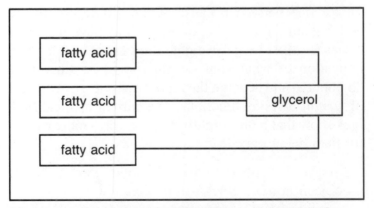

Figure 2.1 Structure of triglyceride or fat molecule

Fatty acids are classified as saturated or unsaturated depending on the number of hydrogen atoms they contain (appendices A-1 & A-2). The unsaturated fatty acids are further classified as omega-1, omega-2, omega-3 and so on, based on where the first unsaturation appears, counting from the terminal carbon (appendix A-3). Most vegetable sources have omega-6 whereas fish oil contains mainly omega-3 type fatty acids. Such small difference as the omega position is crucial in determining how beneficial or harmful these acids are to the body.

Three unsaturated fatty acids, namely arachidonic, linolenic and linoleic, comprise a group of "essential fatty acids," or vitamin F. A minimum amount of vegetable fat is, therefore, important in the diet to provide an adequate supply of these essential fatty acids since the body cannot synthesize them. The minimum dietary requirement is that 1 percent of the total calories in adults and 4 percent total calories in children should be provided by these essential fatty acids. These requirements are easily fulfilled in our daily diets.

The essential fatty acids perform several vital functions such as controlling plaque formation and blood pressure and promoting the body's defense against cancer and infections. The deficiency of essential fatty acids in the body results in retarded body growth, scaly or broken skin and excessive water loss from the body.

The physical and chemical properties of fats determine health hazards. One such property is the liquidity of the fat at room temperature. Saturated fats appear solid at room temperature (or have high freezing point), whereas unsaturated fats generally stay liquid at room temperature. If unsaturated oils are hydrogenated, such as in the prepartion of maragarine, the oil turns solid. As a rule of thumb, liquid fats are less hazardous to health than solid fats.

The omega position, in unsaturated fats, has significant effect on the freezing characterstics. Generally, omega-3 acids freeze at much lower temperature than other omega acids giving the oils containing these acids different characteristics (table 2.1).

TABLE 2.1

FREEZING TEMPERATURE AND SATURATION OF OILS

Oil	Freezing Temp. (°F)	% Saturation
Palm Oil	95 (s)	47%
Butterfat	90 (s)	43%
Coconut Oil	77 (s)	92%
Body fat	59 (s)	36%
Peanut Oil	37	15%
Cottonseed Oil	30	18%
Olive Oil	21	10%
Sesame	21	14%
Soybean	1	13%
Castor Oil	0	3%
Corn Oil	-4	14%
Linseed Oil	-11	3%
Fish Oil	-103	10%

s = solid at room temperature

THE LIPIDS

Fats in the blood are comprised of triglycerides, fatty acids and several other "fat-like" chemicals such as cholesterol, some hormones and vitamins, all of which are collectively termed LIPIDS. The lipids, because of their immiscibility with blood, cannot stay suspended in it any more than a tablespoonful of oil added to a glass of water would. Therefore, to provide

mixing of lipids in the aqueous blood, the body coats
the fatty substances with water soluble proteins making
them into shape of round balls (figure 2.2), within
which are contained triglycerides, cholesterol, phospholipids such as lecithin and a variety of other water
insoluble chemical forms.

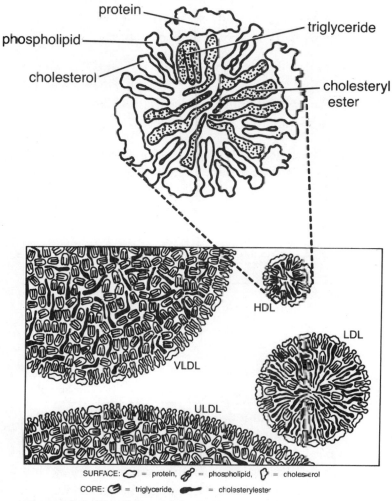

Figure 2.2 The lipoprotein balls in the blood

These fatty balls with a water miscible exterior, called lipoproteins, stay dispersed in the blood and are carried around to wherever they may be needed to supply fat, hormones and vitamins. The percentage of proteins in the lipoproteins, which ranges from 1 to 99, determines how heavy these fatty balls are (appendix A-4) compared to water and what their size is. The heavier balls, called high density lipids are of smaller diameter because of their compact nature.

Generally, the low density lipids contain large quantities of triglycerides and cholesterol and are much more harmful in causing blocking of arteries. This concept will be elaborated on in later chapters.

The concentration of lipids in the blood of healthy individuals varies considerably (table 2.2). It is important to know when your blood becomes "fattier" or shows too high a proportion of the wrong type of lipids.

TABLE 2.2

LIPIDS OF BLOOD, MG/100 ML

Lipid	Mean	Range
Triglycerides	143	80-180
Phospholipids	215	123-390
Lecithin		50-200
Total cholesterol	200	107-320
Free		26-106
Free fatty acids	12	6-16
TOTAL	**570**	**360-820**

Lipids in the blood pose a serious threat to health, causing blocking of arteries, stroke and even cancer. It is, therefore, important to monitor them closely. The following chapter examines the actions of lipids and how they can be modified to ensure better health.

3
THE EICOSANOID POWER

"Power tends to corrupt and absolute power corrupts absolutely."

Lord Action, letter to Mandell Creighton, April 5, 1887

Dietary fat, besides providing energy to the body, controls several vital functions such as circulation, immune system and flexibility of body membranes and cells by converting to hormone-like chemicals in the body called EICOSANOIDS. The eicosanoids are highly potent chemicals produced only in minute quantities by the body cells whenever and wherever they are needed; they cannot be stored in the body. Eicosanoids are composed of about a dozen compounds whose importance has been discovered only in the last 10 to 15 years. According to Dr. William E. Lands, the famous University of Illinois biochemist, whose book, "Fish and Human Health," has just been published by Academic Press, "Eicosanoids are how the cells chatter back and forth with each other." Many eicosanoids have opposing effects and by creating different quantities of these eicosanoids, the body maintains a wonderful balance in its various functions. Many diseases such as heart attack, stroke, cancer, migraine, arthritis, hypertension are now attributed to an imbalance in the production of eicosanoids.

Eicosanoids are mainly formed in the body by arachidonic acid (AA), an omega-6 fatty acid found in vegetable oils. Other omega-6 and some omega-3 fatty acids first convert to AA and thus indirectly contribute to production of eicosanoids. Eicosanoids are also synthesized by omega-3 fatty acids found in fish. However, eicosanoids synthesized from omega-3 acids are distinct from eicosanoids synthesized from omega-6 fatty acids. And it is this difference in the activity of the two types of eicosanoids that makes fish so good for our health.

The effects of eicosanoids range from regulation of blood pressure to causing abortion (table 3.1, appendix A-5).

TABLE 3.1

GENERAL EFFECTS OF EICOSANOIDS

- adrenal gland function
- insulin release
- movement of calcium from bones
- blood clotting
- blood pressure
- action of drugs used in arthritis, high blood pressure and water retention in body
- food digestion
- immune system: resistance to diseases, cancer, infections
- uterine contractions: pregnancy/delivery/abortion

Eicosanoids are divided into two families: the prostaglandins (PGs), which are made by an enzyme called cyclooxygenase; and the leukotrienes, which are made by an enzyme called lipooxygenase (fig. 3.1). Both families stimulate inflammation and contraction of muscles. Some drugs act by blocking cyclooxygenase enzyme so that PGs are not formed. For example, aspirin is recommended to reduce risk of heart disease because of its blocking of PG formation.

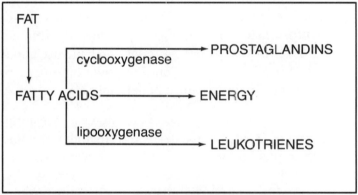

Figure 3.1 Eicosanoid formation from fatty acids

HARNESSING EICOSANOID POWER

The body cells can synthesize 10,000 times more eicosanoids than they normally need; so, the body has tremendous power to control its functions but this power also corrupts. Any outside influence such as diet, tension, smoke, etc., can cause the body to "explode" with eicosanoids, resulting in many diseases. Many techniques can be used to keep the eicosanoid factory operating at a low efficiency level to avert the risk of disease. These techniques are based on either reducing conversion of AA to PGs by blocking the cyclooxygenase enzyme or by reducing supply of AA, an omega-6 fatty acid in the diet.

BENEFITS AND DANGERS OF VEGETABLE OILS

Since all types omega-6 acids convert to AA and thereby contribute to synthesis of eicosanoids, any dietary source of omega-6 acids will aggravate this condition. Unfortunately, it is almost impossible to eliminate omega-6 acids since they are contained in just about all type of foods. However, cutting down on omega-6-rich cooking oils is certainly beneficial.

The most logical approach is to increase consumption of omega-3 fatty acids, derived from both vegetable and fish, replacing omega-6 acids. Unfortunately, very few vegetable sources are rich in omega-3 acids. The best vegetable sources of omega-3 acids are linseed, rapeseed and soybean oils. However, the type of omega-3 acids in vegetable oils is different from those found in fish or other marine sources. The vegetable omega-3 acids are much less beneficial to health than the omega-3 acids derived from fish.

FISH COUNTERACTS THE EFFECTS OF VEGETABLE OILS

The theory which describes how fish proves beneficial to the body is called the "2:3" theory. The body produces two types of prostaglandins (PGs), a group of eicosanoids (appendix A-5): the series-2 and the series-3 PGs. Vegetable oils, rich in omega-6 fatty acids produce more of series-2 PGs, whereas omega-3 fatty acids found in fish produce the series-3 PGs. Higher concentration of series-2 PGs is associated with heart disease, hypertension and stroke. The series-3 PGs, when present in higher concentration, block the harmful effects of series-2 PGs.

The series-2 and series-3 PGs differ in their chemical structure only minutely; the series-3 compounds have an additional pair of hydrogens missing. The fish fatty acids such as EPA produce only the series-3 PGs and, if present in large quantities, tip the balance of PGs to series-3 type in the blood.

Therefore, one of the most relevant element of blood chemistry is the ratio of omega-3 to omega-6 fatty acid. This ratio is several hundred times higher in the Eskimos than in the Western population explaining the resistance of the Eskimos to many diseases so common to the West.

Another beneficial effect of omega-3 acids is related to increased concentration of leukotrienes in the body. High concentration of omega-3 acids in the blood blocks conversion of omega-6 acids to PGs and forces them to convert to leukotrienes, which improves the immune system of body resulting in increased resistance to infections and cancer.

Now that we have seen that unsaturated fat, so highly touted for its beneficial effects, is, in fact, no better than saturated fat, we will examine, in the following chapters, in further detail, how fish counteracts the effects of both.

4

THE AFFAIRS
OF THE HEART

"The heart asks pleasure first,
And then, excuse from pain
And then, those little anodynes
That deaden suffering.
And then, to go to sleep;
And then, if it should be
The will of its Inquisitor,
The liberty to die."

EMILY DICKINSON, Poems. Pt. i. No. 9

Of all the vital organs in our body, the heart is most extolled. Just imagine what the world would be like, if poets and playwrights, lovers and the beloved had no heart to dwell on. Consider the following:

My heart sank when I saw her first;
It terrifies the cockles of my heart;
Eat your heart out America;
No sky is heavy if the heart be light;
Every heart hath its own ache;
An innocent heart is a brittle thing;

A gen'rous heart repairs a sland'rous tongue;
The incense of the heart may rise;
Ye whose hearts are fresh and simple;
Create in me a clean heart, O'God;
A good heart's worth gold;
Soul of fibre and heart of oak;
The hearts that dare are quick to feel;
A gentle heart is tied with an easy thread;
A small heart has small desires;
That which cometh from the heart will go to the heart;
That heart I will give to thee;
A faithless heart betrays the head unsound;
A good heart is better than all the heads in the world;
Some heart once pregnant with celestial fire;
Heartburn;
Heartbeat of America;
And let me wring your heart;
I will wear my heart upon my sleeve;
My heart is ever at your service;
Hearty appetite;
A heart once broken cannot be mended;
My heart bleeds.

Romantic cliches aside, the ailing heart causes more troubles in life and is more to blame for death than any other organ of our body. One out of every four Americans has an ailing heart or blocked arteries, precipitating three heart attacks and one stroke every minute. Half of all deaths in this country are attributed to heart ailments, ranking them second only to respiratory diseases in terms of days-off bed disability but first in terms of the economic cost. The estimated cost for 1986: a hearty 100 billion dollars. Fortunately, the "epidemic" of cardiovascular diseases is on the downgrade in the U.S., having peaked in the 1950s when they accounted for 55 percent of all deaths compared to the current 50 percent. This decline, albeit small, is not a worldwide phenomenon; many European and Asian countries show substantial increase in heart diseases.

Cardiovascular diseases comprise several diverse ailments such as hypertension, stroke, and blocking of arteries. Whereas hypertension or elevated blood pressure can be easily detected in its early stages, atherosclerosis develops secretly in various parts of the body (such as in the arteries supplying blood to the heart and brain) over several decades before the plaques break off, causing hemorrhage and blockage of the arteries. The symptoms of atherosclerosis appear suddenly in the form of heart attack, sudden death, angina, or stroke.

The general hardening of the arteries or arterioslcerosis is another serious disease which causes hypertension and atherosclerosis. Whereas high blood pressure is defined as readings above 160/95 range, the damage due to elevated pressure begins at much lower levels. For example, a healthy 35-years-old man has twice as high a risk of dying if his blood pressure rises from 120/80 to 142/90 and two and a half times more chance of death if the pressure rises to 152/95.

Given the history and the havoc of heart disease, man has long been motivated to search for a cure; none has been found but he did discover that whereas the cures are elusive, the prevention is not. If you can work your way out of the causative factors (table 4.1), you are home safe.

TABLE 4.1

IDENTIFICATION OF HIGH RISK FOR HEART DISEASES

DO YOU:
- suffer from hypertension?
- get easily agitated?
- drink coffee, tea or alcohol excessively?
- eat a lot of red meat?
- like fried foods?
- count yourself among those who have had an open heart surgery?
- feel shortness of breath?
- have sedentary habits?
- smoke?
- have diabetes, hypothyroidism, kidney disease?
- have obesity?
- have a family history of heart disease?
- find it difficult to enjoy a vacation?
- drive to work more than five miles each way?
- get bothered by little matters?
- think you are a pessimist?
- have a sweet tooth?
- hate exercise?

5

PLAQUE ON THE WALL

"My soul is full of longing
For the secret of the sea
And the heart of the great ocean
Sends a thrilling pulse through me."

LONGFELLOW, The Secret of the Sea.

Plaque on the wall of your arteries present no happy picture at all. Essential body nutrition is supplied by the blood flowing through the arteries. The blocking of arteries that nourish the heart results in angina pains, heart attacks and eventually death. Plaque on the wall of brain arteries causes stroke and if plaques grow in the arteries of the limb, blood circulation is severely restricted to various parts of the body.

The incidence of plaque formation is steadily rising in the younger Western population, due principally to the modern lifestyle and diet. The disease itself, however, is not modern; the Egyptian mummies, several thousand years old, show extensive blocking of the arteries. Today, just about all of us have some plaques on our walls; only half of us will survive it.

WHY DO ARTERIES GET BLOCKED?

The many miles of arteries in our body are frequently damaged and blocked for reasons which vary from our diet to our personality (table 5.1).

TABLE 5.1

REASONS FOR BLOCKAGE OF ARTERIES

- Physical damage to arteries
- High fat concentration in the blood
- High clotting activity in the blood
- Old age—fragility of arteries
- Diseases: hypertension, diabetes etc.
- Hormones produced in stress
- Cigarette smoking
- Genetic effects
- Immune system deficiencies
- Free radicals, such as from rancid fats
- Deficiency of vitamins such as B-6
- Reduced antioxidant levels (A, C, E, Bs)
- High insulin levels due to sucrose in food
- Reduced levels of selenium and zinc

Physical damage to the arteries is the most common starting point for plaque formation. The arteries are continuously damaged as some 1.5 gallons of blood flows through them every minute at high pressure. Just imagine, by the time you reach age 40 your heart has pumped about 30 million gallons of blood through your fragile arteries. Given this kind of stress and considering the chemically reactive nature of blood, even copper or steel plumbing would give out, so why not the fragile arteries?

Once damage is reported in any artery, the body goes into motion to repair it immediately. The repair process consists of calling upon the help of several blood components, especially the platelets and the red and white blood cells to form a quick plug at the site of damage, the whole process taking only a few minutes to complete. You have experienced an analogous process when you bruised or received cuts on the skin.

The clotting process is our best defense against bleeding. However, unless checked quickly after repairs, the clots will continue to grow and block arteries. To assure that the clotting and constriction of arteries stops when repairs are completed, the body has an elaborate control mechanism, whereby the arteries produce chemicals to counteract the clotting action. However, if the clotting process is strong or its control defective, large plaques are formed in the arteries precipitating angina pains, heart attacks and strokes.

Excessive clotting activity is a result of the neurotic state of the body's defense systems engendered by our modern lifestyle. If arteries are continuously damaged due to stress, cigarette smoke, carbon monoxide, diet or a host of other causes, the body stays in an alert stage of defense and any assault, albeit small, is handled head on and in a flagrant manner. It is quite obvious that our lifestyle keeps the body in a state of alert and tension most of the time.

Another causative factor for atherosclerosis is the free radicals floating in the body. Diets high in free radicals such as charbroiled foods and rotten cooking oil should, therefore, be avoided. The free radicals are highly charged molecules produced, for example, when oils or fats become rancid or undergo oxidation. Several nutrients such as vegetables, minerals such as selenium and zinc and vitamins such as A, C, E, B-1 and B-6, prevent the formation and dissipation of free radicals in the body.

MECHANISM OF PLAQUE FORMATION

Formation of plaques in the arteries is a complex process that takes years to complete. The process begins with a rupture of the artery either due to physical damage or to accumulation of fat, mainly the low density type, in the lining of the arteries. This fat forms deposits, or atheromas, which is Greek for porridge. These atheromas grow steadily and destroy the lining of the artery, whose repair results in the formation of plaques (figures 5.1 and 5.2).

The repair of the arteries involves summoning blood platelets to the site (there are about 1-2 billion of these particles floating in our blood) to release a chemical messenger, thromboxane, which induces two actions to prevent blood loss: one is the clumping of platelets and other blood cells and second, the narrowing of the opening of the arteries. To keep this process under control, the arterial walls release another messenger, prostacycline, to counteract the effect of thromboxane (details in appendix A-6). Both thromboxane and prostacycline have very short lifespans and last only a few minutes after they are released at the site of damage. The body must, therefore, be always ready to synthesize these prostaglandins on demand. The raw material for these chemical messengers is the unsaturated fatty acids, more specifically, arachidonic acid, supplied in our food.

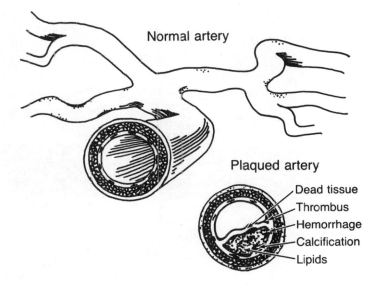

Figure 5.1 Plaque formation

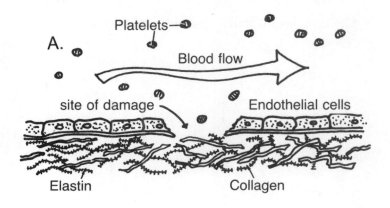

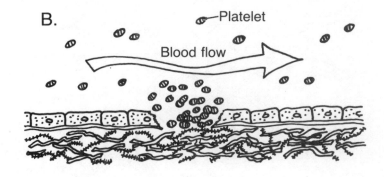

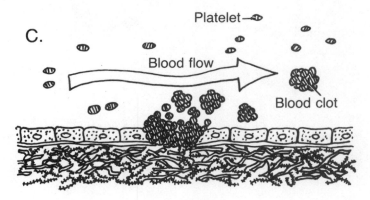

Figure 5.2 Clot formation

There are two types of PGs formed, the type 2 from omega-6 fatty acids and the type-3 from omega-3 fatty acids. Whichever type of acid is present in higher quantity will provide its own type of PGs since the conversion of fatty acids to PGs is a competitive process where both types of fatty acids compete for the limited amount of enzyme available in the blood. If the concentration of omega-6 type acids is high in blood, as a result of high consumption of vegetable fats, the type-2 PGs formed in excess will accelerate the process of plaque formation.

Saturated fatty acids, on the other hand, cause heart disease by promoting the initial infiltration of arterial walls which causes arterial damage. Therefore, both saturated and unsaturated fats in our blood are involved in causing atherosclerosis. It is difficult to assess which type of fatty acid is more harmful. In recent years, we have reduced the use saturated fats, but increased the use of vegetable oils, a situation which is no better than if we had continued the use of saturated fats. *This is contrary to the popular belief that only saturated fats need to be avoided in our diets but it certainly explains why the incidence of atherosclerosis has not declined in proportion to the reduced saturated fat intake. The key to reducing incidence of atherosclerosis is to reduce all types of fats, not just the saturated fat.*

Most vegetable oils, rich in unsaturated fat, increase the concentration of arachidonic acid (AA), an omega-6 fatty acid, in the body which results in increased production of eicosanoids which elevate blood pressure, reduce the body's ability to fight off infections, especially cancer, and increase the tendency of saturated fat to collect in the arteries causing heart attacks and strokes. These findings shatter the myth that only people who consume large quantities of saturated fats have high risk of heart disease.

Similarly, stress and smoking also cause plaque formation by increasing the production of hormones such as epinephrine and norepinephrine, which are related to the clotting activity of the blood. It has been estimated that if all Americans stopped smoking, we would save at least 170 thousand lives per year, most highly productive men and women at the peak of their careers. It is encouraging that since 1965, the number of male smokers has fallen by 30 percent, but unfortunate that women smokers have declined by only 14 percent. On an average, there is about a 35 percent decline in the per capita consumption of all types of tobacco in this country. Yet, it is not enough. It is ironic that our government spends millions of dollars to prevent deaths from traffic accidents, but very little to save four times as many lives by discouraging the use of tobacco products.

The sex of an individual also determines his or her susceptibility to heart disease. Generally, younger women are relatively free from heart disease because of the protective effects of female hormones. However, when they reach the age of menopause their immunity is lost as a result of reduced female hormones. The male hormones, on the other hand, increase the blocking of arteries by keeping the clotting process hyperactive. This is a result of evolutionary adaptation when man, facing uncertain elements, was victim of the "fight or flight" syndrome. Even today, stress from everyday chores is sufficient to keep the body's defense systems alert and hyperactive. As women have increasingly taken on the role of breadwinners, their risk of heart disease has risen significantly. As we age, the risk of dying of heart disease increases because our arteries harden, become more brittle and lose their resilience, all of which contribute to increased blocking of arteries.

The fact that each individual responds differently to the multitude of factors which govern blocking of arteries, proves that genes too play a role. Our genes determine how resistant we are to heart ailments; genes control the vulnerability of arteries to physical damage, infiltration by blood fats, and the delicate balance of the chemical messengers involved in plaque formation; genes also control our stressability, fat metabolism and hypertension. However, at times, genes have been a catchall excuse for effects which defy scientific explanation.

The biggest genetic myth was recently shattered when the statistics on atherosclerosis was summarized for the world population. Earlier observations from postmortem reports on soldiers killed in recent wars had shown massive atherosclerosis in the Americans as compared to the Chinese and Japanese soldiers. This was attributed to genetic immunity in certain populations and coincided with the belief that the Japanese and Chinese have genetic immunity to heart diseases. New studies show that the Japanese who settled in Hawaii lost immunity to heart disease once they adopted the Western lifestyle and diet, disproving the early myth.

Another interesting observation compares Eskimos and Finns. Although both belong to the same Mongolian race, the Finns show a much higher rate of heart disease than do the Eskimos.

HOW TO AVOID BLOCKED ARTERIES?

Having understood the factors that cause our heart to go on the blink, we should be able to devise concrete means to counteract them. Most of these measures can be classified as either dietary or nondietary. The nondietary measures comprise mainly the use of drugs, physical exercise, reducing smoking and avoiding stress to keep our hearts healthy. However, the need for these measures can be significantly reduced and other factors, such as genetic tendencies and aging counteracted, if the dietary measures are properly instituted.

The dietary measures consist mainly of selecting food which least promotes plaque formation: the choice of saturated vs. unsaturated fats in our diet.

CHOICE OF SATURATED VS. UNSATURATED FATS

Reducing the use of saturated fats, advice that has been constantly repeated, is of prime importance. Plaque formation is either caused by high fat concentration in the blood or the transformation of fat into plaque when an artery is ruptured. The type of fat which is most dangerous in this regard is the low and ultra low density lipids which are mainly made up of triglycerides, some cholesterol and plasma proteins. The concentration of these lipoproteins is decreased if we reduce the use of saturated fats.

The major contribution to our saturated fat (appendix A-1) comes from the cooking fat, and the meat and dairy products in our diet. It is relatively easy to cut down saturated fat coming from cooking oils. Whatever fat is present in our food first passes through our blood and if it is solid on our plate, chances are it will quickly turn solid in our blood also. The rule of thumb is that if a cooking fat solidifies at room temperature or clouds in the refrigerator, it is not good for health. Just remember if it does not solidify at room temperature, it has less than 20 percent saturated fat.

Reducing consumption of saturated fat is, however, not an easy task because of the concentration/quantity relationship of fatty foods. The quantity of saturated fat consumed depends not only on the concentration of saturated fat in the food but also on the quantity of food consumed; for example, a common serving of french fried potatoes has less saturated fat than a routine single serving of yogurt or milk. What is worse, therefore, french fries or yogurt?

Of course, there are additional considerations such as vitamins and minerals supplied by milk which are not provided by french fries. However, in a planned dietary program these supplements can be provided easily by other foods. The goal should be to reduce consumption of all saturated foods (table 5.2). It is interesting to note that, with few exceptions, most saturated fat foods provide about same quantity of saturated fat whether they are low or high in it because of the amount we eat.

TABLE 5.2

SATURATED FAT IN COMMON FOODS

Food	%	Av. Serving (Gm)
Yogurt	1	2
Milk, low fat	1	2
whole	3	5
Fried chicken	2	1.5
French fries	3	1.2
Pizza	3	2
Avocado	3	6
Shrimp, fried	3	2
Sardines, canned	3.5	3
Eggs	3.5	1.5
Almonds	4	5
Walnuts	5	6
Beef, ground	5	6
Veal	5	4
Ice cream	7	9
Pie crust	8	4
Pumpkin seed	8	12
Safflower oil	9	1.3
Hot dog	10	6
Potato chips	11	2
Pork	12	9
Corn oil	12	2
Margarine	14	1
Olive oil	14	2
Mayonnaise	14	2
Peanut oil	16	3
Bacon	17	2.5
Candy, chocolate	20	5
Cheese	22	5
Veg. shortening	25	3
Coconut	31	4
Palm oil	40	8
Lard	40	5
Butter	51	2.5
Coconut oil	95	?

Given the bad effects of saturated fats on our health, unsaturated fats, derived from vegetable sources, have become fats of choice during the past 20-30 years. These fats solidify at much lower temperature and are generally preferred because of their perceived lesser harmful effects. This theory has recently been refuted. Omega-6 fatty acids in vegetable fats increase the tendency to form plaques exacerbating the effects of the saturated fats (appendix A-6). There are also other deleterious effects of omega-6 acids which will be discussed later in this book. The current consensus is that vegetable oils are equally as harmful as saturated fats and the worst combination is when both types of fats are taken in excess.

It has become increasingly clear that we should avoid all types of fats, vegetable and saturated animal, but the type of food Americans prefer makes this next to impossible. There are too many sources of fat, based on cooking methods, that most us may not even be aware of (table 5.3).

TABLE 5.3

HIDDEN SOURCES OF FAT

Food	Grams of fat
Meat, Fish, Poultry (3 ounce serving)	
Pan fried	7
Basted	7
Marinated with oil	7
Breaded and fried	15
Vegetables (per cup)	
Stir-fried	5
Seasoned	5
Breaded and fried	10
French fried (per 20 fries)	20

Eggs (each)	
Fried	5
Scrambled	all fat added
Salads (per cup)	
Potato, macaroni	10
Slaw or fruit	40
Meat or egg	40
Sauces (per tablespoon)	
Gravy	8
White sauce	8
Tartar	8

Just when attempts to reduce fat in our diet may seem like a lost cause, comes the good news that not all types of fats are bad. The fat in fish can be highly beneficial to the body. The omega-3 fatty acids, available only in fish, counteract the effects of both the saturated and unsaturated fats in our diet and restore the body systems damaged by these undesirable components of our diet.

THE UNIQUE FISH FAT

The effect of a fish diet on blood chemistry is related to its consumption in large quantities. For example, a recent study reported from Japan compared the blood levels of omega-3 fatty acids in people living in Kawazu, a fishing village, with that of the population in the neighboring Kamagaya, a predominantly farming village. The report showed that when fish is the preferred diet (250 G/day), the ratio of omega-3 over omega-6 fatty acids in the blood remained high, which is the key to reducing risk of heart disease. In this study, the fishing population had only one-third the clotting activity compared to the farming-village population. The incidence of heart disease was proportionally smaller in the fishing population as well.

Additional studies in Denmark have shown that whereas more than half of the deaths there are attributed to heart disease, less than eight percent of Eskimos deaths are a result of heart problems. A comparison of the diet of the Danes and the Eskimos (appendix A-7) quickly solves this discrepancy.

The Eskimos take twice as much cholesterol per day as the Danes, but their consumption of omega-3 fats is about 5 times higher than the Danes. Of great importance in our diet is the "P/S" ratio, the polyunsaturated to saturated fat ratio, which is about four times higher in the Eskimo diet compared to the Western diets.

Omega-3 acids exert two distinct actions in the body, a physical action due to their low freezing points and oily nature, and a chemical action altering the type of chemical messengers produced in the body.

THE PHYSICAL ACTION

Fish sailing in the cold arctic water remain supple and flexible because of high concentrations of omega-3 fatty acids, which keep the membranes of the cells from freezing; in other words, the low freezing property of these fatty acids maintains the "fluidity" of the body membranes at low temperatures. Thus, the cellular membranes of anyone consuming large quantities of fish will have higher "fluidity", reducing the rigidity of arteries and lowering the blood pressure, both of which contribute to reduce blocking of arteries.

The, high concentration of omega-3 fatty acids in the body also makes the red blood cells more flexible and deformable, allowing them to move readily and reach oxygen starved tissues which improves the utilization of energy in the body.

THE CHEMICAL ACTION

Omega-3 fatty acids produce PGs such as thromboxane and prostacycline, similar in chemical structure to the ones produced by the omega-6 fatty acids but with different effects in the body. The thromboxane causes clotting and narrowing of arteries whereas prostacycline counteracts these effects. The thromboxane formed from omega-3 acids does not have the clotting ability and therefore the net effect is that fish fatty acids prolong bleeding, reduce blood clotting and significantly reduce plaque formation, all by soothing the hyperactive clotting mechanism of the body (appendix A-6).

The effectiveness of a diet rich in omega-3 acids is measured by how it alters the ratio of omega-3 to omega-6 fatty acids in the blood. A high ratio means either a higher concentration of omega-3 or a lower concentration of omega-6 acids. Keeping this ratio high results in a substantial reduction in plaque formation. This ratio in the Eskimos is four times higher than in the Japanese population and 70 times higher than the U.S. and European populations. The overall incidence of heart disease among these populations can be correlated to this ratio directly. It is easy to understand why this ratio, and not the concentration of either types of fatty acids in blood, is important. The omega-3 and omega-6 fatty acids compete for conversion to the chemical messengers responsible for plaque formation; hence, whichever type of fatty acid is present in higher quantity with respect to the other prevails. The goal is to have a high concentration of omega-3 and low concentration of omega-6 acids in blood.

It is important to know that all of the effects of omega-3 fatty acids are of transient nature and if one stops eating fish or taking supplements of fish oil, the platelet counts and their ability to stick to the wall return to normal.

A similar mechanism applies when aspirin acts to reduce plaque formation, except that this effect is much more prolonged. Aspirin destroys the enzymes which cause conversion of fatty acids to prostaglandins, whereas in the case of omega-3 fatty acids, they are only temporarily blocked. A fish diet combined with aspirin, will prove tremendously effective in prolonging bleeding times while reducing the stickiness of platelets to cell walls.

The phenomenal effects of a fish diet or omega-3 acids, on reducing the incidence of heart disease should be appreciated by all those who are at high risk for these diseases.

6

LEAVING THE FAT OUT

*"Many more people by gluttony are slain
Than in battle or in fight, or with other pain."*

**UNKNOWN,
Dialogues of Creatures, p. 128. (c. 1535)**

Food does more than satisfy hunger. Food brings disease; it cures disease. Food makes us happy; it makes us sad. Food sustains life and it invites death. Essential to our body, food, can also be more lethal than any other offering of Nature to man. Not all types of food are bad; it is that touch of grease that kills. The human blood is already pretty greasy, adding any more grease to it by eating fat-rich food is like adding insult to injury.

The level of fat in our blood is determined by many factors (table 6.1), the foremost being the diet; it does not take very long for the bite of hot dog or fried chicken to be felt on your heart. All types of saturated fats convert in our body to "bad lipids." The unsaturated fat, touted as a healthy substitute for satuated fat, is equally bad when it comes to causing plaques in the arteries. So, it does not matter, what type of food you eat; if it is fatty, it's going to hurt.

TABLE 6.1

FACTORS CONTROLLING FAT IN THE BLOOD

Factors Increasing	Factors Decreasing
Saturated fats	Unsaturated fats
High cholesterol diet	Cholesterol free diet
Male hormones	Female hormones
Age	Thyroid hormones
Stress hormones	Genetic makeup
Genetic makeup	Aerobic exercise

The American love affair with fat is a heavy one. In the year 1985, we consumed over 15 billion pounds of fats in preparing our foods alone (table 6.2). It is difficult to estimate how many more billion pounds of fats were consumed as food itself, but it is substantial.

TABLE 6.2

COOKING FATS USED BY AMERICANS (1985)

Cooking Fat	Pounds, billion
vegetable oil	6.3
shortening	4.8
margarine	2.5
butter	0.8
lard	0.8

There is a general misconception about the role of saturated vs. unsaturated fats in our body. The current consensus is that neither one is better than the other. The only way out of blocking our arteries is to avoid all fats, saturated or unsaturated.

Next to our diet, but directly related to it, is obesity which is now classified by the U.S. government as a disease and not merely a condition. The more we weigh, the more our body feels it needs to keep stores of fats to provide energy and the vicious cycle continues. As soon as you start to reduce your weight, blood fats decline immediately.

Our age has an important bearing on the amount of fat present in our body. With each passing year we lose muscles and become less lean causing the level of fat in the blood to rise.

Sex hormones and the hormones released when we are under stress have significant effect on blood fat. Male hormones increase the blood fat while female hormones keep it down. No wonder women have much lower incidence of heart disease. The effect of stress hormones such as epinephrine is about equally deleterious in both men and women.

Finally, genes are implicated as a causative factor for a rise in blood fat when we cannot explain it otherwise.

HOW TO REDUCE BLOOD FATS

Diets rich in vegetable oils reduce the floating levels of fats in our blood by reducing the supply of the raw material needed to synthesize these fats. In this regard, the polyunsaturated fats are much more effective than the monounsaturated fats, which have only neutral or

mild ability to reduce fats or cholesterol in the blood.
In Chapter 2, the degree of saturation of various cooking
oils was listed in table 2.1. A quick way of telling which
oil has more polyunsaturated fatty acids is by their
melting or freezing points. Highly unsaturated oils have
lower freezing points and do not cloud at room temperature or in the refrigerator. Fish oil, for example, freezes
at − 70 degrees, while butterfat freezes at 32 degrees.

The advice to reduce intake of saturated fat has
been well received by the American public as reflected
in substantial reduction in the use of dairy products and
animal fats (table 6.3).

TABLE 6.3

DECLINE IN THE USE OF SATURATED FATS
DURING 1977-86

Fat source	Decreased by
Milk	16%
Cream	18%
Butter	38%
Egg	18%
Animal fats	40%

The significant decline in the use of saturated fat
has resulted in an average reduction of about 5 percent
in the blood fats, a small, but encouraging change.
However, the incidence of heart disease, instead of
declining proportionally, has risen during this time, a
perplexing statistic. The reason for this discrepancy has
recently been discovered. What has happened in recent

years is that although Americans have reduced the consumption of saturated fat, they have, at the same time, more than compensated for it in the increased consumption of unsaturated fats.

Long-term studies from England show that from 1935 to 1960, the Britons increased their omega-6 fat consumption two-fold resulting in a seven-fold increase in deaths from heart disease. In subsequent years, from 1960 to 1975, when the use of omega-6 fats did not change, the risk of death from heart disease also remained unchanged.

Therefore, it really didn't matter that we reduced the saturated fats in our diet. It turns out that the unsaturated vegetable fats weren't such a good substitute after all. Omega-6 fatty acids have now been implicated in gall stone formation, decreased resistance to diseases, increased incidence of cancer and reduced breathing of heart and other muscles in addition to the effects on plaque formation described earlier. These indictments make vegetable oils just as, or perhaps more, undesirable than the saturated fats.

Another dangerous aspect of the use of unsaturated fat is its chemical instability. Unlike saturated fats, the unsaturated fats and oils quickly break down under heat or upon exposure to air, resulting in rancidity (the odor) and conversion of fat molecules to free radicals, which increase plaque formation and cause cancer. The fat ground with meat is particularly susceptible to breakdown and cooking food on an open fire simply makes it more carcinogenic and worse for the heart.

EFFECT OF FISH DIET ON BLOOD FATS

Just like vegetable oils, but two to five times more effectively, the fish diet reduces the floating levels of fat in the blood. However, the nature of this change is different. In 1983, Dr. William Harris and his associates compared salmon oil with vegetable oil and found that the vegetable oil diet lowers the cholesterol levels slightly, while salmon oil not only decreases the most dangerous fats such as triglycerides and low density lipids, it also elevates the good cholesterol (table 6.4). This effect of fish diets is most helpful in preventing plaque formation.

TABLE 6.4

CHANGES IN BLOOD FAT DUE TO FISH DIET

Fat	Changed by
Cholesterol	10-20% (reduced)
Triglycerides	30-60% (reduced)
HDL	5-10% (INCREASED)

It is now possible to explain why Eskimos and others who consume large quantities of fish (about 25 times more than an average American) have reduced fat in their blood despite their fat-rich food.

Americans do not eat large quantities of fish for many reasons, not the least of which is the wide choice of foods available to them. Few Eskimos would pass up a piping hot sausage pizza if delivery could be made to their igloos.

Fish also fell into disfavor due to the bad publicity given some types of fish which are labeled fatty and, therefore, forbidden in the same vein as other saturated fats. Fish are labeled fatty because of an erroneous analysis of their fat content reported many years ago. Current reports from the U.S. Department of Agriculture list crab and lobster roughly equal to the dark meat of chicken in cholesterol but with much lower concentrations of other fats. Shrimp has slightly higher cholesterol content, but only moderately so. The "oily fish" such as salmon, mackerel, bluefish, lake trout, sardine, and herring have only about one-fifth to one-half the average fat content of the leanest beef. Shell fish such as shrimp, lobster, oysters, scallops, clams and crab are also low in fat. There really is no fatty fish which can be harmful.

Recent studies conducted at the Oregon Health Science University show that diets high in fatty fish, such as salmon, actually lower blood cholesterol and triglycerides. Even shell fish, taken on a daily basis, either reduces the blood cholesterol or has no effect on total blood fat content. Fish of all types are, therefore, beneficial in preventing atherosclerosis and its free use is recommended.

Omega-3 oils in fish more than compensate for any undesirable effects they may have. To stay lean, we must keep the omega-3 fatty acid content in our bodies high. Unfortunately, the body cannot store these acids and we must continue eating fish, which is how fish do it themselves. In a recent study by Dr. S. M. Boggio, it was shown that when rainbow trout are fed swine fat, the omega-3 content of trout decreases significantly. Fish eating other fish or algae rich in omega-3 fatty acids have high body content of omega-3 oils. Ever heard of fish needing a bypass?

If you are still not convinced, read the October 7, 1986 issue of the New England Journal of Medicine, which reports that pigs fed high fat diets avoided heart disease if their diets were supplemented with fish oil. If it is good for pigs why not for those of us who love to pigout? Fish helps undo what other diets do to you. It will let you live despite yourself.

Currently, Americans are taking more than 50 percent of their calories as fats—half of which are saturated fats. The unsaturated fats in our diet are mostly of the monounsaturated type, which is closer in properties to saturated fat. The polyunsaturated fats account for about 15 percent of all calories, of which only one-tenth is of omega-3 type. And even the type of omega-3 fat we take is mostly of the type which is not beneficial to the heart. This situation must be changed, if we are to have any hope of living long.

7
NO MORE HYPERTENSION

"Life is like a scrambled egg."

DON MARQUIS, Frustration.

Frustration has a lot of company. Tension, frustration and the rigors of the modern day life are the prime causes of hypertension, which can be a cause or a result of blocked arteries. Hypertension kills by causing failure of heart, kidneys and brain. If your blood pressure is higher than 160/95, you have a 5-30 times higher risk of coronary atherosclerosis (blocking of heart arteries) and stroke.

All factors which cause atherosclerosis also cause hypertension. However, the factor most directly related to hypertension is stress. Stress is caused whenever your moods change, you cry or laugh, you worry or feel excited, you feel loved or hated, you achieve some goals or lose some. The effects of stress are cumulative and you need to evaluate periodically how you are

managing your life or your life is managing you. Here's
a quick test to find out how you score (table 7.1).

TABLE 7.1

DO IT YOURSELF TEST FOR STRESS TESTING

Rank	Event	Score
1	Death of spouse	1000
2	Divorce	750
3	Separation	650
4	Jail sentence	600
5	Death in family	590
6	Illness or injury	525
7	Marriage	500
8	Lost job	475
9	Marital reconciliation	450
10	Retirement	450
11	Pregnancy	400
12	Sexual difficulties	395
13	Substantial change in net worth	375
14	Death of a close friend	375
15	Change to different line of work	350
16	Change in arguments with spouse	350
17	Large mortgage	325
18	Mortgage foreclosure	300
19	Change in work responsibilities	295
20	Child leaving home	295
21	Trouble with in-laws	290
22	Outstanding personal achievement	285
23	Begin or end school	260
24	Wife begins or stops working	260
25	Trouble with boss	240
26	Change in residence, school, or church	200
27	Small mortgage or loan	175
28	Change in sleeping habits or family get together	150
29	Vacation	125
30	Religious holidays	110
31	Traffic violations	100

HOW TO SCORE: Add all scores for events that took place during the past 12 months. Scores up to 1500, you are doing fine; between 1500-3000, you have moderate stress, watch out; scores over 3000, you need help now—buy fish today.

Through the process of evolution, our body has become accustomed to handling stress by exhibiting a "fight or flight" syndrome. When under stress, our body releases hormones which increase heart rate and blood pressure to supply more blood and oxygen to tissues to combat the cause of tension. There is also a simultaneous increase in the sugar and fat content of blood. Therefore, the net effect of stress is that our blood gets sweeter, fattier, thicker and "clottier," all of these causing an increased tendency to deposit fat in the arteries.

Therefore, the best possible way to avoid heart disease is to avoid stress, advice which cannot be easily followed. However, you can learn to control your body's response to stress. A study reported in October 1986 by the American Heart Association states that by adopting a less competitive lifestyle you can reduce the risk of heart disease by more than 50 percent. For example, by simply letting others finish talking without interrupting them may add several years to your life. The famous personality classification of type A (hyperactive) or B (calm), should be reviewed to see if you can cultivate the B profile.

Role Of Fish In Reducing Hypertension

A simpler and more immediate means of reducing hypertension is to add fish to your diet. The Eskimos and the Japanese maintain much lower blood pressure than the Americans because of the concentration of omega-3 fatty acids in their blood. Recalling the discussion in an earlier chapter, omega-3 acids dilate arteries and keep blood flowing smoothly; vegetable-oil-derived omega-6 acids, on the other hand, constrict arteries and raise blood pressure.

Omega-3 acids also have an effect on the elasticity of blood vessels. With age, and as a result of continued tension, our arteries harden (arteriosclerosis), therefore, cannot relieve increased pressure effectively by expanding. Omega-3 fatty acids keep membranes of body cells, and as a result our arteries, more supple and flexible. The high concentration of omega-3 acids in the walls of red blood cells makes them more easily penetrable to deeper tissue, providing better oxygenation of all body tissues. Therefore, the overall effect of fish diet is to reduce hypertension and allow freer breathing of body tissues. The increased breathing of tissues also reduces formation of free radicals, which are implicated in blockage of arteries, especially in the brain (stroke).

The January, 1987 issue of the Prevention Magazine includes an impressive testimony by Charles D. Neal of Carbondale, Illinois. Neal had a chronic problem of hypertension. He asked his doctor to monitor him on a fish oil therapy. The results were startling (table 7.2).

TABLE 7.2

FISH OILS LOWER BLOOD PRESSURE: A CLINICAL TRIAL

Parameter	Change in 8 weeks
Systolic pressure	180 to 138
Cholesterol levels	253 to 195
Triglyceride levels	150 to 104

Neal's doctor said, after examining him eight weeks later, "The outcome was unbelievable. If I hadn't supervised the experiment myself, I would not have believed the results."

The beneficial effects of fish can be substantially increased if you also adopt other recommendations to reduce the incidence of hypertension and plaque formation (table 7.3).

TABLE 7.3

RECOMMENDATIONS TO REDUCE RISK OF HYPERTENSION.

- maintain ideal body weight
- reduce fat in your food by half
- reduce or eliminate use of dairy products
- avoid egg yolks and organ meats
- be moderate in your lifestyle
- give up smoking
- eat as much and as many types of fish as possible
- eat meats of all types sparingly
- exercise regularly, especially aerobic type
- keep smiling
- drive at 55 mph
- don't interrupt others talking
- accept your spouse's refusal of sex gracefully
- try finishing second or third at times

- cross the bridge when you come to it—do not worry
- learn to use time effectively
- rationalize events

8
THE CHOLESTEROL MYTH

*"The anatomy of any myth
is the anatomy of the men
who believed in it and suffered by it."*

**MURRAY KEMPTON,
"A Prelude," Part of Our time (1955)**

Cholesterol is almost a household word and we all know how bad cholesterol is for our health. Or do we? The public bias against cholesterol is well established and hardly anyone would believe me if I said that the bad effects of cholesterol have been blown out of proportion.

The fact is, cholesterol is a very useful fat, serving as a precursor to various essential hormones and vitamins. The cholesterol in our skin prevents us from absorbing many dangerous chemicals in our polluted environment and also helps restore the water in our body to prevent dehydration. Cholesterol also acts as a potent antioxidant, protecting the body from cancer-causing free radicals. Finding anything else floating in the blood half as good as cholesterol would be quite a task.

There is no denying that cholesterol is associated with heart disease but not in the way we generally believe. Not knowing what cholesterol is and does, can make our efforts to reduce risk of heart disease less meaningful.

Cholesterol is found abundantly in foods (table 8.1). The highest concentration of cholesterol occurs in the organ meats and egg yolk. Organs such as liver, kidney and brain are extremely high in cholesterol. Most other foods have somewhat comparable levels of cholesterol.

TABLE 8.1

CHOLESTEROL CONTENT OF COMMON FOODS

Food	Cholesterol, mg/100 G
Yogurt	6
Milk	14
Cookies	55
Fish (most)	25-70
Meat, poultry	70
Turkey	80
Veal	90
Cheese	90
Giblets	200
Butter	230
Kidneys	375
Eggs	500
Brain	2,100

Unlike the essential fatty acids and proteins, cholesterol need not be supplemented in our diets since it is synthesized by the body (about 1.5 grams per day, if no cholesterol is supplied in the diet). Normally we have about 10 grams of cholesterol (in various forms) floating in our blood at all times. To control the level of cholesterol, our body increases or decreases production of cholesterol; however, there are limitations in the body's ability to adjust levels of cholesterol. It takes about five days for a 50 percent turnover or consumption of floating cholesterol. When diets supply excessive cholesterol, the body cuts down its cholesterol production units, and the levels of cholesterol rise only if body cannot dispose off excessive cholesterol.

Therefore, taking cholesterol-free diets may not always lower cholesterol levels in the blood. In fact, some cholesterol in our diet is recommended to keep cholesterol producing systems in the body working at a lower efficiency. The American Heart Association recommends no more than 300 mg of cholesterol per day for men and 225 mg per day for women. So, there is no reason to use those expensive "cholesterol-free" bland foods.

Before we plan to reduce floating cholesterol, we must recognize why the body needs cholesterol in the first place. One such need is the antioxidant, or cancer-protection action of cholesterol. If these needs can be satisifed by alternate means, the body will reduce floating levels of cholesterol itself. Generally, if the level of antioxidants such as vitamins A, E, C and some Bs is sufficient in the body, cholesterol levels will be reduced.

CHOLESTEROL AND BLOCKING OF ARTERIES

The connection between cholesterol and plaque formation and hardening of the arteries is a well established one. High levels of cholesterol cause heart attacks–but not in all individuals. It is easy to make cholesterol a scapegoat but cholesterol is not harmful until combined with other fatty elements in the blood, at which time it demonstrates its vicious characteristics. However, before we get into these fine deliberations, let's examine the evidence connecting cholesterol to heart disease.

The most conclusive study regarding the role of cholesterol in heart disease was released in 1984 by The U.S. Lipid Research Trials, which showed that a 14 percent decrease in the blood cholesterol levels resulted in a 19 percent reduction in the incidence of heart attacks. This reduction was achieved by using a drug called cholestyramine, which helped remove cholesterol from the diet by bonding to it and making it unabsorbable. Another study in 1978 showed that a 9 percent decrease in the cholesterol level resulted in a 25 percent decrease in the incidence of nonfatal heart attacks but no reduction of fatal heart attacks. In 1981, a study from Norway showed that a simple modification in diet resulted in a 40 percent reduction in deaths from coronary heart disease.

These studies demonstrated that there is some effect on heart disease by cholesterol but it is not consistent and reproducible. What is interesting here is that the studies which concentrated in removing cholesterol from the diet using drugs had lesser success than the study where simple diet modifications were introduced.

A low-fat diet would reduce not only cholesterol but also many other types of fats such as omega-6 acids, etc. So, there is sufficient evidence now which suggests that more than just cholesterol is the culprit in our diets.

It is now widely accepted that low density lipids (LDL) are responsible for damage to arteries and heart; whereas, the high density lipids (HDL) prevent formation of plaques. Cholesterol of both types is found in the blood. There is sufficient evidence in the medical journals to prove the beneficial effects of HDL. For example, women experience fewer heart attacks than men; one of the several reasons for this is the higher levels of HDL in women. Exactly how the HDL and LDL differ in the formation of plaque is not fully understood. It is suspected, however, that the LDL, being larger in size (figure 2.2), do not pass through the arteries readily and get trapped, causing infiltration of the arteries (figure 5.1). The HDLs, which are smaller but heavier particles, can easily pass through and can even help "lubricate" the flow of blood fats, much like rolling a heavy object on a ball bearing.

So, the culprit in our blood is not only cholesterol but other types of fats as well; even cholesterol can be good when it is part of the HDL. Therefore our goal should be to increase, not decrease, the fat levels in blood which are of high density type and decrease only the LDL. The risk of heart disease increases dramatically when the concentration of high density cholesterol decreases (table 8.2).

TABLE 8.2

RISK OF HEART DISEASE AND HDL LEVELS

	% Cholesterol as HDL	
Risk	Men	Women
One-half	25	33
Average	20	22
Two-times	11	14
Three-times	4	8

Slight increase in HDL, such as from 20 percent to 25 percent reduces the risk of heart disease by 50 percent for men; women, who are more resistant to heart disease require greater change, from 22 to 33 percent to cut the risk of heart disease to the same degree. When it comes to increased risk due to lowering of HDL or increase in total cholesterol, men can cope with more total cholesterol than women. A three-fold increase in risk to heart disease develops when HDL levels drop to eight percent of all cholesterol in blood for women and four percent for men.

The risk of heart disease should, therefore, be measured in terms of the ratio of total cholesterol to HDL rather than the total cholesterol. For example, you may have above average level of cholesterol but if a substantial percentage of it is present as HDL then it is better than having a lower total cholesterol. Therefore, you should try to increase your HDL instead of worrying too much about the total cholesterol. One way to do it is by exercise.

Physical aerobic exercise increases the concentration of HDL and reduces the concentration of LDL. Joggers have considerably higher levels of HDL, which depends more on the distance covered rather than on the speed. The current trend toward walking instead of jogging is definitely in the right direction.

No drug is currently available to selectively reduce LDL or increase HDL levels. When diet modifications are used, they most likely alter the total fat levels rather than a particular type. One diet component that has significant effect on blood fat levels is the polyunsaturated vegetable oils, which reduce both the LDL and HDL levels and therefore the ratio of HDL may not change (table 8.2).

Several gimmicks are also on the market, such as the use of lecithin which promises to reduce cholesterol and the risk of heart disease. None of these work; some can even be very harmful since they can upset the balance of various chemicals in the blood.

FISH AND CHOLESTEROL

The only dietary tool for reducing blood fats, especially the LDL, while maintaining high levels of HDL, is the use of fish. An interesting study, in this regard, was reported in 1984, when 100 subjects were given two teaspoons of fish oil twice daily with food. After 24 months the blood fats were measured to reveal a most startling favorable change in the blood fats (table 8.3).

TABLE 8.3

EFFECT OF FISH DIET ON BLOOD CHEMISTRY

Parameter	Change in 24 months	
Triglycerides	reduced by	41%
Cholesterol	reduced by	5%
HDL levels	*increased* by	15%
Platelets	reduced by	7%

The fish diet not only reduced the dangerous trigly-ceride and cholesterol levels but increased the beneficial HDL level, a feat never before achieved by diet or drugs. Also altered, the study found, was the platelet count and their activity, both responsible for causing plaques to form. This study established, beyond any doubt, the beneficial effect of fish in bringing the most favorable changes in the blood chemistry. We could not ask for a better medicine, if one existed, to combat heart disease.

A diet of fish or supplementary fish oils are also highly recommended for those who consume high cholesterol diets habitually. An interesting study was reported by Dr. Paul Nestel in 1986, in which subjects consuming large quantities of egg yolk showed no change in their cholesterol level if their diet was supple-mented with fish oil. Therefore, the therapeutic value of fish in reducing cholesterol levels is firmly estab-lished.

Critics of the above recommendation state that not all types of fish can be eaten in large quantities because of their high cholesterol content. This misconception must be clarified. Information in Chapter 2, showed that there is no fish, regardless of its habitat, which can be labeled high in cholesterol. For example, shellfish such as shrimp, lobster and crab, the most commonly criticized fish, have much lower cholesterol than generally assumed.

Shell fish got a bad name several years ago when an erroneous report was made about their cholesterol content. The mistake was that cholesterol and like substances were totaled and reported as cholesterol. We now find oysters, clams and scallops to have about 50 percent less cholesterol than previously reported, so there is no reason why people can't eat them.

LIQUID CHOLESTEROL

Several new studies on the effects of fish on heart disease were presented at the annual meeting of the American Heart Association in November 1986. One examined the nature of the fatty deposits formed when omega-3 acid concentration is high in the blood. The fatty deposits or atheroma are more "liquid" and have lesser ability to clog arteries when fish is eaten frequently. The low freezing quality and lubricating ability of omega-3 acids is responsible for this change in the nature of fatty deposits.

MISTER FIXX

Jogging might be labeled the number-one pastime for health-conscious Americans and Jim Fixx was certainly its chief advocate. His book, *Running*, headed the best seller list for many months. The man practiced what he preached. He was a slender and lean man who ran every day and kept his cholesterol, triglyceride and other fat levels at below normal levels, but he died of a sudden heart attack with massive atherosclerosis while running. He died young and the nation was shocked. Had we understood the relationship between the floating cholesterol or fats and atherosclerosis and heart attacks we would have been less surprised.

Nothing is a simple as it seems and certainly not the stark advice to keep cholesterol levels low to help prevent heart attacks. Not only is it the cholesterol but a lot of other lipids in the blood which contribute to heart disease. It is the tendency of these lipids to accumulate that causes atherosclerosis and not just their mere existence in the blood. And what causes them to form a deposit is highly individualistic. Many people can survive with high concentrations of cholesterol in the blood without ever developing atherosclerosis, and a good number of us will develop atherosclerosis while keeping our blood cholesterol levels way below normal according to population averages.

Cholesterol has become almost a dirty word, yet the truth is, cholesterol is an essential chemical for body growth which can also prevent heart attacks and atherosclerosis. Unfortunately, the consumer industry is often too quick to capitalize on these "emerging" scientific concepts, causing us to go from one extreme to the other. You see all around you, products which are "low in cholesterol," "free of cholesterol" and which have "no cholesterol." You may be consuming less cholesterol, but this is not necessarily safe for your heart.

If a diet promotes plaque formation, it is immaterial whether it is a low or high cholesterol diet. For example, we know that vegetable oils help reduce cholesterol levels, but do they reduce incidence of atherosclerosis and heart attack? Probably not. A large number of processed foods appear safe to a naive consumer because they are free of cholesterol, but are they less likely to cause atherosclerosis? Probably not.

9

READ THY LABEL

*"He who knows not and
knows not he knows not:
he is a fool—shun him."*

**DARIUS, the PERSIAN.
Spectator, 11 Aug, 1894**

Now that we know all about good and bad fats, good and bad cholesterol, good and bad omegas, all we need to do is avoid the bad things in our food to prolong our lives. It is, however, easier said than done. First, what is good for health may not taste good and even if we develop a taste for it, we cannot be assured that we are getting what we asked for. Sounds confusing? Well, it is, and then some.

The food industry regulations in America are in such state of chaos that it is all but impossible to make an intelligent selection of food based on the information available to the consumer. On the one hand there is the processed food manufacturer who is trying to push a lot of sugar, chemical additives, saturated fat and poor quality proteins under the cloak of a confusing label and on the other hand there is the health food industry which is inviting you to eat bushes and berries.

If in the midst of all this the consumer gets confused, that is precisely the goal of the marketing geniuses. Do you really believe that five-year-old Mikey knows which cereal is good for him and unless you buy it immediately he will throw a temper tantrum in the middle of the grocery store aisle? Or how about an eighteen-year-old who insists on organically grown vegetables laced with raw manure at three times the price for an identical product grown normally and available in your neighborhood grocery store?

In a nutshell, the consumer is in big trouble when it comes to proper nutrition, mainly because he is poorly informed about what he is eating. But it is not entirely the fault of the food industry. Few consumers bother to read and understand the labels on their food products. Therefore, guarantees of proper nutrition must begin with attempts to "read thy label."

The U.S. government has enacted regulations by which all packaged foods must display labels with complete information about their contents. The contents must be listed in the decreasing order of their quantity in the package. You can estimate the quantity of a specific ingredient from the position it appears in the list. But beware of the language used on the labels. This is very carefully, and often very cleverly, designed by people who have spent their lifetime studying rhetoric and jargon. For example, a clever label begins with the following statement: "May contain one or more of . . ." followed by a long list of vegetable oils, animal fats, lard, etc. Most consumers pick up the first few words quickly and assume that this product is probably made of vegetable oil while, in fact, it may be made mostly of saturated fat. It is easy to understand why such deceptions are necessary, from a manufacturer's view point. Given a long list of possible ingredients he will choose saturated fat, which is the cheapest and gives the longest shelf life to products.

THE COCONUT CONNECTION

An excellent example of deceptive labeling is that of nondairy creamers, where the label clearly reads "may contain one or more of the following . . . coconut oil, safflower oil, etc." Nondairy creamers are full of coconut oil, which is cheap and helps improve the taste and appearance of the product. But coconut oil is also one of the richest sources of saturated fat So whenever you come across a statement like, "may contain one or more . . ." assume the worst.

Coconut oil and meat are extremely harmful and should always be avoided. The most convincing evidence to support this recommendation was unveiled at the November 1986 meeting of the American Heart Association held in Dallas. Dr. Harry Davis reported that monkeys fed a diet high in coconut oil had over 79 percent of their heart arteries blocked. Other monkeys fed lower levels of coconut oil experienced almost one-half the incidence of coronary artery disease. Here again the use of fish oil helped reduce the deleterious effect of coconut oil diet. The plaques found in the arteries of monkeys fed fish oil appeared less likely to cause heart attack than the plaque seen in monkeys who were given no fish oil.

Coconut is perhaps the most widely used component of packaged foods. You may touch these foods, but only with a 10-foot pole.

POLYUNSATURATED OR JUST UNSATURATED

When it comes to reporting how much saturated fat there is in a product, the industry does a superb job of confusing the whole issue. Do you know how much saturated fat is present in margarine boldly labeled, "Made from 100 percent corn oil?"

When it comes to shortening or margarine, the following principles should be kept in mind:

Not all shortening is of vegetable origin.

Not all vegetable shortening is unsaturated.

Not all unsaturated shortening is polyunsaturated.

Not all polyunsaturated shortening is good for health.

In selecting shortening, your goal should be to choose one that has more polyunsaturated oils than saturated oils. The monounsaturated oils, though classified as unsaturated, are closer to saturated fats in their effects on the body than the polyunsaturated oils. You must always insist on oils which have more polyunsaturated fat and less saturated fat as reflected in their P/S (polyunsaturated/saturated) ratio (table 9.1).

TABLE 9.1

POLYUNSATURATED TO SATURATED RATIO OF SHORTENINGS

Shortening	P/S Ratio*
Coconut oil	0.02
Palm kernel oil	0.02
Beef tallow	0.09
Mutton fat	0.19
Lard	0.30
Chicken fat	0.54
Olive oil	0.63
Peanut oil	1.78
Cottonseed oil	1.94
Soybean oil	3.84
Corn oil	4.58
Sunflower oil	4.60
Safflower oil	7.85

* Polyunsaturated/saturated fat

Note that except for coconut or palm oil, all animal fats have much higher saturated fat content. The vegetable oils high in polyunsaturated components are quite cheap: why not use sunflower or safflower oil for your daily cooking? Remember, only the P/S ratio tells you the amount of polyunsaturated fat in a product. Insist on finding out the polyunsaturated fat content and not the total unsaturated fat in your foods. If the P/S information is not listed on the label, chances are it is high in saturated fat. If you are still not sure, write to the manufacturer of your favorite product.

THE CASE AGAINST MARGARINE

Food labels on margarine and similar artificially processed foods like imitation whipped cream are always deceptive. Their singular purpose is to pass off saturated fat as unsaturated fat by labeling it, "partially hydrogenated," which means that the fat in the product has been chemically changed to make it more saturated. Hydrogenation of vegetable oils results in raising the melting point of oil, giving it a solid consistency.

The degree of hydrogenation determines how solid the product turns out to be but rarely does any label state the extent of hydrogenation. Instead, they all call it "partial" hydrogenation, which may include anything up to 99 percent, without being legally deceptive. So if you see a label saying the product is made of 100 percent vegetable oil, but partially hydrogenated, assume you are getting a lot of saturated fat.

The chemical process of converting unsaturated oils into saturated fat involves the use of highly reactive metallic catalysts, whose residues may be found in the finished product. These residues are highly reactive and can be injurious to health.

It should be remembered that saturated fat is cheap and stable, since saturation removes the unsaturation sites which react with oxygen to make oils rancid or foul smelling. But the process of hydrogenation defeats the purpose of using a polyunsaturated oil. You do not get the same effect of lowering body fats from margarine as you get from polyunsaturated vegetable oils. The saturated fat consumed as margarine has characteristics similar to the fat in butter or lard.

Using margarine, however, creates a situation which is much more hazardous than the use of natural saturated fats. The process of artificial saturation changes the physical and chemical nature of oils (appendix A-8) so that they are not easily used by the body for energy purposes; they elevate blood cholesterol and triglycerides and accumulate in heart muscles and weaken them. Therefore, the use of margarine not only loads you up with saturated fat but in a form which is alien to the body and can be more dangerous than natural fat.

The case against margarine and all other imitation dairy products is a strong one. When you use butter, you know what you are getting into or what is getting into you, but when you use margarine you are at the mercy of a chemist. Butter has only twice as much saturated fat as margarine so why not use butter but cut the quantities you use in half.

THE HOLY COW

Milk and dairy products contribute more fat to our body than all other sources put together. The health hazards of cow's milk are enough to fill a book but we will review them briefly here. Milk is a mixture of lactose, fat and casein (table 9.2) all of which cause heart disease or disturbances of the gastrointestinal tract. However, the possible contaminants in milk make it doubly undesirable. The fat soluble nature of milk makes it an ideal storage tank for all the cow eats, inhales or produces as refuse in her body. The problem with milk is that it reflects the nature of our environment in a more concentrated form. If our air is not clean, our milk supply won't be. Our environment, and, as a result fodder, is often heavily contaminated and we get it all back when we drink milk. The common contaminants of milk are pesticides, herbicides, carcinogens,

antibiotics, hormones, fertilizers, etc. If this were a
man-made product, would you buy it? The vitamins
and minerals in the milk can easily be obtained from
alternate sources, so why expose your body to heart
disease, cancer and a variety of other complications?

TABLE 9.2

COMPOSITION OF MILK

Component	Percentage
Water	87.50
Lactose	4.70
Fat	3.75
Casein	2.90
Ash	0.75
Other proteins	0.40
Vitamins, minerals	traces

There is a direct correlation worldwide between
per capita milk consumption and the risk of diseases
from the chemical and microbiologic contamination in
milk. Other hazards of milk are allergies and intolerance
due to lactose and proteins in milk.

Milk substitutes, with the same beneficial properties
and less objectionable properties are casein hydroly-
sates, soy formulas and goat and ewe milk. Selection
of an appropriate alternate must be based on caloric
and growth requirements.

Combining milk and peanut butter, a common lunch
for millions of American children, is also very dangerous. The peanut butter is full of arachidonic acid,
omega-6 fatty acid, which directly converts to the PGs

which cause all the problems of the arteries and heart. On top of that, the milk adds fat, which increases blockage of arteries, increases the number of fat cells in the body and stores carcinogenic chemicals. There can be no more devastating combination of foods for children.

THE FINAL COMMANDMENT

There is really only one goal in selecting foods; to avoid all types of fats where possible. Currently, we take 50 percent of all of our calories as fats, a figure which can easily be cut in half without sacrificing the greasy taste we cherish so much. We can start by becoming intelligent readers of our food labels.

10

THE MALIGNANT CELL

*"He who has a thousand friends
has not a friend to spare,
And he who has one enemy
shall meet him everywhere."*

**ALI-Ibn-ABU-TALIB (7th c.), quoted
in Emerson's Conduct of Life, 7.**

There are billions of molecules in the body and if only one goes haywire, it can take the entire body with it. Cancer, the dreaded disease, is of the body's own making and is responsible for one out of four deaths in this country. Cancer occurs when a single body cell becomes unresponsive to the normal controls of the body and the neighboring cells. This results in expansion and growth of similar carcinogenic cells. The malignant (harmful) tumor in contrast to the benign (harmless) tumor, invades the local tissue and spreads to different parts of the body (metastasis), destroying everything in sight.

What causes a body cell to turn cancerous is not clearly understood. However, many sources which contribute to cancer have been identified (table 10.1).

TABLE 10.1

MAJOR CAUSES OF CANCER

Source	% all cancer
Cigarette smoking	35
Genetic factors Radiation Air pollution Occupational exposures	10-20
Viruses	5-10
Unknown causes	50-60

The unknown causes, which account for the majority of cancer cases, make this disease especially dreadful and mysterious. Sporadic observations show:

• Mormons, who shun coffee, tea and alcohol, have a much lower incidence of cancer.

• Sexual activity may help prevent prostrate cancer, the theory being that sex hormones built up during abstinence can reduce the immunity of prostate cells to cancerous growth.

• Rancid fats are possible causative agents for colon and breast cancers.

• Burnt and browned meat and fat are highly carcinogenic.

• Sedentary people contract cancer six times more frequently than the physically active.

• There is a clear link between obesity and breast cancer in women. Cancer patients who weigh less than 140 pounds have a 62 percent survival rate five years after breast surgery, as compared to 49 percent for those patients who are over 140 pounds or overweight according to standard weight height charts.

- A study from Johns Hopkins University School of Medicine states that the cancer survival rate is increased in patients who are able to articulate their feelings of anger, fear, and depression. Patients who talked about their emotions outlived by a margin of three to one those who did not. This may have to do with the hormonal levels when negative feelings are suppressed.

- In the year 1900, mortality due to cancer was only 4 percent of all deaths as compared to 25 percent today. In the year 1900, more people died of injuries than from cancer.

- High fiber and low fat diets provide protection against many types of cancers (For additional information on this topic you may call 1-800-4-CANCER, The National Cancer Institute, and ask for their free booklet on nutrition and cancer or write, NCI, P. O. Box K, Bethesda, Maryland 20814. Another excellent reading reference is "Dietary Guidelines for Americans" provided free by the U.S. government. Write to Consumer Information Center, Dept. 622 N, Pueblo, Colorado 81009).

Our environment is full of reasons why body cells should become cancerous. It is surprising that, despite this, only one out of four people develop cancer. Immunity to cancer is attributed to the elaborate defense mechanisms of our body. Cancer cells, being different from normal cells, evoke a protective response causing a rush of fighting blood cells called macrophages, those tiny "Pac-man-like" structures which literally chew up the cancer cells. This is analogous to a blitz at the line of scrimmage during a football game. Any disorder of the body or condition which suppresses the defense system of the body makes us more susceptible to cancer. The majority of cancers of unknown causes can be attributed to this reduced immunity against cancer.

HOW FOOD CAUSES CANCER

Since drug treatment of cancer is not very effective, it would seem more important to prevent the disease from beginning in the first place and with food targeted in five of the nine observations above, it would certainly be prudent to look to our diets.

The food components play opposite roles: they may be carcinogenic themselves or may prevent other components of food from causing cancer. For example, cruciferous vegetables such as cabbage are recommended since they reduce the carcinogens in our diets.

TABLE 10.2

SOURCES OF CARCINOGENS IN FOOD

Chemical contamination: food processing and packaging, preservatives such as nitrates, environmental contamination.

Thermal decomposition: charbroiling, breakdown of proteins and fats in cooking.

Food spoilage: rancid oils, decomposed foods.

Most of the identified carcinogens (table 10.2) can be avoided by careful food preparation and storage. Several food additives such as the antioxidants (chemicals which keep fats from turning rancid such as BHA and BHT) and free radical quenchers (chemicals such as vitamin E which deactivate the highly reactive molecules) are often recommended in cancer prevention therapies. The value of these therapies remains questionable.

Recently, investigators have begun looking into relationships between fat in our diet and cancer. Fat causes cancer by two mechanisms. First, most chemical carcinogens are of the fat soluble type and the more fat we consume, the greater our chance of being exposed to these carcinogens. Second, unsaturated fats reduce the immunity our body has to cancer. Vegetable oils cause cancer by:

- Breaking down to carcinogens (rancid oils are high in carcinogens);

- Increasing concentration of cancer promoting PGs, and

- Reducing body immunity to cancer growth.

It is ironic that the increased consumption of vegetable oils to lower cholesterol levels and heart disease has resulted in substantially increased risks to several types of cancers.

FISH TO THE RESCUE AGAIN

Fish contains high concentrations of vitamin A & D, which have been associated with cancer prevention, the theory being that these vitamins inactivate the cancer-causing free radicals from the body.

Recently, the role of omega-3 fatty acids in the prevention of cancer has been explained. This theory is best summarized in the Catalog of Federal Domestic Assistance No. 13.293, Cancer Cause and Prevention Research by the Public Health Service of the U.S. government. In this document, and in scores of scientific publications, it has been observed that the risk of developing cancer at certain sites such as the breast, colon, prostate, pancreas, endometrium and ovary can be reduced by supplementing the diet with fish.

Fish consumption has been correlated with a lower incidence of breast cancer in Greenland and Japan. Greenland Eskimos, whose caloric intake is almost 70 percent fat (mostly whale and fish), have almost no incidence of breast cancer, and in Japan, where the breast cancer rate is the second lowest in the world, 50 percent of the fat intake comes from fish. The total fat intake in Japan is almost 20 percent compared to 40-50 percent in America. However, not all types of cancers have low occurrence in the Eskimos and the Japanese. This finding further supports the theory that diet and environment have significant connection with carcinogenicity. As a result, the overall incidence of cancer in Greenland Eskimos is only slightly lower than the Western population. Future studies must identify the sources of other carcinogens in the diet and life of Eskimos to enable us to better utilize components of their diet in preventing the types of cancers most prevalent in our society.

How omega-3 fatty acids in fish help prevent cancer is a complex mechanism (appendix A-9 and table 10.3). A simple explanation is that omega-3 fatty acids reduce the carcinogenicity of vegetable oils and boost the body defense system against cancerous cells.

TABLE 10.3

HOW FISH PREVENT CANCER

Reduce cancer promoting PGs (such as PGE_2).

Restore body's defense against cancer:

* increased activity of macrophages, the "Pac-Mans" of human body,

* increased concentration of arginase, the "bullets" in macrophages.

* increased production of leukotrienes.

* increase vitamins which inactivate cancer-causing free radicals.

The free-radical fighting properties of fish have additional effects since free radicals are also implicated in aging, heart disease, arthritis, cataracts, senility, dandruff and bruises. Therefore, a fish diet not only protects us from heart disease and hypertension but possibly from cancer and many other diseases.

However, eating fish does not induce any permanent change in the body chemistry. The protective effects of fish last only as long as you continue to eat it. For example, we find that the Japanese who settled in Hawaii and changed their fish-eating habits, increased their risk of cancer. Similarly, the Eskimos who settled in the Netherlands have shown just about same risk of developing cancer as the native Danish population. The transient effect of fish on our body is an added advantage since it allows us to avert any long-term side effects of eating fish or taking fish oil supplements.

Despite the many questions that remain to be

answered, there are a number of thing we can do to reduce the risk of developing cancer (table 10.4).

TABLE 10.4

RECOMMENDATIONS TO REDUCE INCIDENCE OF CANCER

Avoid obesity.

Reduce dietary fat, both saturated and unsaturated.

Eat Fish.

Eat more high fiber foods, such as whole grain cereals, fruits and vegetables.

Include foods rich in vitamins A, C and other natural antioxidants in the daily diet.

Include cruciferous vegetables, such as cabbage, broccoli, Brussels sprouts, kholrabi, and cauliflower in the diet.

Be moderate in consumption of alcoholic beverages.

Be moderate in consumption of salt-cured, smoked, and nitrite-cured foods.

Avoid ultraviolet light exposure such as sun tanning, natural or artificial.

Avoid unnecessary exposure to chemicals.

Stop smoking or chewing tobacco.

Avoid exposure to any types of smoke.

Exercise regularly.

Reduce tension.

Reduce consumption of charbroiled or burnt foods.

11

DISEASES OF THEIR OWN ACCORD

*"Diseases of their own accord
But cures come difficult and hard."*

**Samuel Butler, The Weakness and
Misery of Man, 1. 82.**

The biggest culprit when it comes to causing many serious diseases is the body itself. When an outside "element" enters the body, the immune system of body gets to work to eliminate it; however, in the aftermath of the war with the foreign "element," the body is left with chemicals that bring symptoms of asthma, arthritis, lupus, psoriasis, multiple sclerosis, diabetes, rejection of transplants and many other still unexplained diseases.

An overzealous body defense system, at times, gets so active that it starts fighting its own cells and so the diseases of immune system are truly of their own accord. There really is no way to prevent these diseases and only symptomatic treatments are used to suppress body's immune system by using potent drugs like steroids.

However, like so many other secrets of the sea, comes a panacea for, perhaps, the most perplexing of all human ailments—the body's desire to self destruct.

Omega-3 fatty acids also control disorders of the body immune system as evidenced by Eskimos, who rarely show any of these diseases. The eicosanoids formed from omega-3 acids reduce the activity of the body immune system; however, this containment of the immune system is highly selective and does not affect the body's ability to fight-off infections and cancer. If these eicosanoids were to depress the immune functions indiscriminately, the body would quickly succumb to various diseases as has happened with AIDS (acquired immune deficiency syndrome), for which no treatment has so far been found. The selective action of omega-3 on the body immune system actually enhances the infection-fighting ability of the body.

ARTHRITIS

Inflammation of tissues is caused by various blood cells, such as monocytes and platelets, sticking to the site of injury and releasing chemicals. Since omega-3 fatty acids reduce the stickiness and chemical reactivity of these cells, inflammation, which results from arthritis and physical injuries, is defused.

Omega-3 acids also alter the types of leukotrienes formed by omega-6 acids which cause inflammation and hypersensitive reactions. Studies conducted at the

Albany Medical College and reported in the September 1986 issue of the Internal Medicine News show extremely beneficial effects of EPA (the omega-3 acid in fish) in treating rheumatoid arthritis. This study observed significant reduction in the number of tender joints in subjects treated with a fish oil for only 14 weeks. Another study reported from the Harvard Medical School on 13 patients showed similar results.

The future of omega-3 fatty acids in treating arthritis and similar ailments is very bright. It should be noted that aspirin, which is the drug of choice for relieving arthritis pain, has a similar action. A combination of aspirin, or other anti-arthritic drugs, with fish oil is a highly effective combination for symptomatic treatment of arthritis.

In addition, omega-3 fatty acids have the ability to make cell membranes more "fluid" thus, in effect, "lubricating" the joints.

ASTHMA AND ALLERGIES

The symptoms of asthma are caused by eicosanoids which fight "foreign" particles in the body or at times its own cells. Eskimos show extremely low incidence of asthma because of altered composition of eicosanoids. However, the fish oil therapy can be beneficial only in the early stages of asthma since once the allergic reaction has been established it is not possible to eliminate it. Eskimos benefit because they take omega-3 rich diets from infancy. Perhaps we need to start teaching our children the value of fish diets in their early years.

Fish oil also reduces the collapse of lungs during severe allergic reactions, as observed in many studies on animals fed high fish oil diets. The question arises whether these fatty acids will have any future role in the development of anti-allergy medicines? It is likely they will.

GRAFTS AND TRANSPLANTS

Patients taking fish oil supplements are more receptive to venous grafts (such as performed in heart bypass surgeries) than those who do not. From the mechanistic point of view, it is entirely plausible to establish the role of omega-3 fatty acids in organ transplants and in the case of cardiac bypass patients. The latter, highly susceptible to blockage of arteries, are perhaps the best target group on which to investigate the long-term effects of omega-3 fatty acids in preventing the recurrence of artery blockage.

Another beneficial effect of fish oil therapy can be drawn from its ability to thin out the blood or prolong the bleeding. Anticoagulant drugs are often prescribed for heart patients. Can omega-3 supplements reduce the need for these drugs? A dietary solution would be preferred over any drug therapy. However, if you are prescribed any anticoagulant drugs such as warfarin, consult your physician before you begin on fish oil supplements or even plan to include more fish in your diet.

MIGRAINE

Anti-immune and vasodilation effects of omega-3 fatty acids relieved migraine pains for patients on high fish oil diets, recent studies have reported. Since migraine pains have a myriad of causes, not all of which may be affected by omega-3 fatty acids. Highly variable effects of fish diet are noted in migraine patients. In one study at the University of Cincinnati, College of Medicine, five out of six sufferers from migraine headches, had fewer, less severe headaches when they took 20 grams of a commercial fish oil preparation in contrast to those on a placebo.

DIABETES

There are three types of diabetes. Type I, also known as Juvenile Diabetes, typically occurs in pre-teen years. These patients do not produce enough insulin to sustain life and must inject themselves regularly with insulin. Type I diabetes also occurs in older people and there need not be a family history of the disease to acquire it. Type I diabetes occurs because the body's overzealous "protector" cells start to chew up the insulin producing cells of the pancreas. It is suggested that omega-3 acids reduce the activity of these "protector" cells and can help control the onset of Type I diabetes. Some drugs which provide the same function must be used for prolonged time and can have their own side effects; the use of diet rich in omega-3 fatty acids is a definitely better alternative to potent drugs.

Type II diabetes typically strikes overweight people who are past 40 and have a strong family history of diabetes. These people produce enough insulin at the beginning of their illness but develop insulin resistance as the disease progresses. Their bodies just do not respond to the insulin secreted by their own body. Type

II diabetics eventually become insulin dependent as the disease progresses and their insulin production slows down or ceases. About 80-90 percent of diabetics have Type II, which is not often insulin dependent.

The third type of diabetes is gestational diabetes, which affects mainly pregnant women during the middle or last trimester but disappears following delivery.

Several beneficial effects of a fish diet have been observed in Type II diabetic patients, who traditionally have a very high death rate from heart diseases. Even short term treatment with concentrated fish oil results in a significant decrease in the blood triglyceride levels and an increase in the HDL levels, a combination highly beneficial to reducing the incidence of blocking of arteries. At the 1986 meeting of the American Diabetes Association, several important findings of the effect of fish oil in treating Type II diabetes were reported. There is also evidence that omega-3 fatty acids directly affect insulin production and sensitivity of body cells to insulin. The low incidence of Type II diabetes in Eskimos may be also be attributed, in addition to their high omega-3 intake, to the low amount of refined carbohydrates in their diets.

LUPUS

Lupus (Systemic lupus erythematosis) is a chronic disease of damaged blood vessels and kidneys. The damage to blood vessels results in high blood pressure and plaque formation leading to heart attacks. The dietary omega-3 fatty acids produce eicosanoids which interfere in the initiation and progression of lupus as observed in Eskimos and others who consume high quantity of omega-3 fats.

MULTIPLE SCLEROSIS

The connection between multiple sclerosis (M.S.) and the body's immune function is not clearly understood but M.S. patients show improvement when given fish oil. Because of the severity of the disease, however, any help in the treatment, albeit rudimentary, should be taken seriously; why not try omega-3 therapy?

12

THE NEW AGE
OF AQUARIUS

"When the moon is in the seventh house
And Jupiter aligns with Mars,
Then peace will guide the planets,
And love will steer the stars;
This is the dawning of the age of Aquarius,
The age of Aquarius."

HAIR (1966). Aquarius

Although some of the ways in which fish prove beneficial to our body have been elucidated, many other applications remain to be discovered. The previous chapters of this book dwelt mainly on the use of fish in averting heart disease, cancer and diseases of the immune system because to date most of the research has been devoted to those areas. However, evidence has started to emerge on the benefits to be gained in treating other ailments.

EFFECTS ON EYE, BRAIN
AND REPRODUCTIVE ORGANS

Omega-3 acids, in particular the DHA, are found in very high concentration in the eye retina, brain, testes and sperm and regardless of the dietary intake of these fatty acids, the levels of DHA are constantly maintained in these specific organs. This constancy of level suggests an important role of DHA in the functioning of these organs.

Within the eye retina, the DHA makes up about 50 percent of the fatty acid content in the specialized membranes which record light. It is not known exactly how DHA helps in the function of eye but its carbon chain length and high degree of unsaturation help create a membrane with high fluidity, flexibility, and permeability, the characteristics necessary for the dynamic behavior of photoreceptor membranes. The DHA-rich membranes also provide for specific transport channels for various enzymes and amino acids, such as taurine, all found essential for membrane integrity and function.

In the brain, where several highly specialized membranes are present, DHA may account for 30-50 percent of the fatty acids. The DHA and other unsaturated fatty acids accumulate in the brain rapidly during pregnancy and immediately after birth. During the last trimester of pregnancy, the brain content of these fatty acids increases three to five times; similar percent increases occur again between birth and 12 weeks of age in the newborn. After birth, newborns are limited in their capacity to synthesize DHA and other acids and remain dependent on dietary sources. The fat in the mother's milk contains these acids in sufficient quantity to provide for their accumulation and brain development. Unfortunately, most synthetic infant formulas provide no DHA or arachidonic acid and as a result these infants have far less DHA in their blood than infants receiving human milk, even when an ample supply of other fatty acids, such as linolenic acid is provided. It is ironic that even the largest manufacturers of infant formula have not addressed this crucial deficiency in their products. What effects this has had on the brain development of millions of infants will never be known, but is it worth the risk?

To date no definite signs of omega-3 fatty acid deficiency have been recorded in humans, but then we may be looking for the wrong signs. The most likely indications of such deficiency will be lack of brain and sight development and inadequacy of the reproductive system, such as infertility. The old wives' tale that fish is brain food has now been upgraded from a tale to a fact.

KIDNEY DISEASES

Several recent studies have shown that omega-3 fatty acids can protect patients from a variety of kidney diseases by promoting body mechanisms similar to those which affect cancer. While still preliminary, these studies are quite promising.

INFECTIONS

It should be obvious to the reader by now that omega-3 fatty acids have almost magical curing properties. Thus, news of a U.S. Patent (Appl 630,732) on the use of dietary supplements rich in fish oil as a protection from or treatment against infections is truly exciting. The patent suggests giving these supplements orally or through the veins to prevent a variety of infections.

OTHER DISEASES

Research is also currently being conducted in the application of fish oils to the treatment of psychiatric disorders, cystic fibrosis, skin diseases, alcoholism, premenstrual tension, etc. All of these studies have sound scientific basis and it is likely that in the near future many therapeutic applications of omega-3 fatty acids will emerge.

BLEEDING TENDENCIES AND OTHER SIDE EFFECTS

Since Eskimos bruise easily and show prolonged bleeding, a fact known for some 500 years, some investigators are concerned about the prolonged bleeding that may result during the use of fish diet or oils. However, according to Dr. Desmond David of R.P. Scherer, the manufacturer of MaxEPA, "People have taken up to 20 (1 gram) capsules per day without any side effects." There is no doubt that fish increases bleeding tendency, but this effect is always temporary and can be reversed quickly. There is no scientific study reported to date where increased bleeding is reported as a serious side effect. However, those on anticoagulant therapy must consult their physicians before taking fish oil supplements or even when eating more fish.

IRRITATION AND ALLERGIC RESPONSE

There are reports of sporadic individual reactions to the consumption of fish oil, especially on an empty stomach. These effects include tightness of the stomach, regurgitation, facial flushing, etc. However, discontinuing the use of fish oil immediately relieves the side effects.

VITAMIN E ABSORPTION

. Another side effect of a high fish diet or fish oil supplements is the reduced absorption of vitamin E. Since vitamin E affects the metabolism of omega-3 fatty acids and the formation of PGs, as well as performing several other essential functions, there is a need to provide vitamin E supplements for those on a high fish diet or on high fish oil supplements. It is also advisable to take vitamin E supplements at times other than when taking fish or fish oil, to avoid any physical or chemical interaction in the absorption of vitamin E.

Future studies on the effect of fish oils are likely to confirm additional benefits as we learn more about how eicosanoids work in our body. We may also discover additional side effects of fish oil as more people start using them. But whatever is known today points to fish oil becoming an ultimate panacea for mankind.

13

TO FISH OR NOT TO FISH?

"Of all the world's enjoyments
That ever valued were.
There's none of our employment
With fishing can compare."

THOMAS D'URFEY,
Pills to Purge Melancholy:
Massaniello: Fisherman's Song.

Given the scientific evidence in the previous chapters, it becomes evident that we must load our bodies with omega-3 fatty acids. This can be accomplished by eating a lot of fish, especially, the fatty kind; by taking those golden pills that contain fish oil; or by going directly to marine algae or weeds to find a supply of omega-3 acids. This chapter examines those choices.

A FAT YOU CAN LOVE

The fat in fish is "good" fat. But not all fish have the same "goodness," or fat content. Fish can be categorized as one of two types—those that store fat in muscles such as mackerel, salmon and herring, and those that store fat inside the body such as cod. In the latter category, not highly recommended, most of the fat is found in the liver, not much of which is eaten. Therefore, a serving of cod or similar fish will not provide any substantial amount of omega-3 fatty acids. Also, cod liver oil has excessive concentrations of vitamins A & D (two teaspoonfuls twice a day is equal to twice the recommended daily allowance of vitamins A & D), which, combined with other sources of vitamin A & D in our diets, can be toxic. The highest fat found in any fish is about 16% compared to 30% in sirloin steak. So the fattiest fish is still leaner than other meats (table 13.1).

TABLE 13.1

FAT CONTENT OF FISH

(INCREASING ORDER IN EACH CATEGORY)

1% or less:
Cod, haddock, northern pike, blue shark, mahimahi, yellow perch, rockfish.

1% to 5%:
Snapper, flounder, walleye, monkfish, Atlantic croaker, pacific pompano, smelt, striped bass, pacific, halibut, yellowfin tuna, brook trout, skipjack tuna, ocean perch, bluefish, barracuda, Atlantic sturgeon, Atlantic halibut, sea catfish, chum salmon, swordfish, channel catfish, pacific mackerel, anchovy, pink salmon.

5% to 10%:
Bonito, Atlantic salmon, rainbow trout, Spanish mackerel, bluefin tuna, cisco, coho salmon, sardine, albacore tuna, sockeye salmon, Atlantic herring, carp, whitefish, lake trout, pompano, pacific herring.

10% to 15%:
Atlantic mackerel, lake sturgeon, butterfish, king salmon, shad, sablefish, American eel, buffalo.

The beneficial effects of fish fat are mainly due to two principal ingredients, eicosapentaenoic acid (EPA) and docosahexaenoic acid (DHA), which comprise about 30 percent of the total oil in fish. The quantity of EPA and DHA is higher in "fatty" fish—the fish living in cold water. The fatty acids in cold water fish are less saturated than the fish in warm or fresh waters. The degree of saturation of fatty acids determines how harmful they are for the heart; this applies to fatty acids derived from fish, as well as those derived from vegetable or animal source.

Keep in mind that when you eat fish, you naturally get more than just the "good" fat. Fish also contain many other saturated or unsaturated fatty acids (appendix A-10), which may be harmful to the body, if fish is eaten frequently.

The choice of fish should depend, besides taste and texture, on the amount of omega-3 acids yielded in proportion to the total calories (tables 13.2, 13.3 and 13.4).

TABLE 13.2

OMEGA-3 CONTENT OF FISH

Fish	% Omega-3
Sockeye salmon	3.0
Albacore tuna	2.3
California bilchard	2.0

Spiny dogfish	2.0
European anchovy	1.9
Coho salmon	1.8
Atlantic mackerel	1.8
Chinook salmon	1.7
Pink salmon	1.5
Anchovy	1.4
Lake trout	1.4
Atlantic salmon	1.4
American eel	1.3
Pacific herring	1.3
Atlantic halibut	1.3
Sablefish	1.2
Bluefin tuna	1.2
Cisco	1.1
Rainbow Trout	1.0
Swordfish	0.9
Striped mullet	0.9
Spanish sardine	0.9
Atlantic herring	0.9
Whiting	0.9
Striped bass	0.7
Yellowfin tuna	0.6
Red Snapper	0.6
Channel catfish	0.6
King Crab	0.6
Pacific halibut	0.5
Carp	0.5
Shrimp	0.5
Ocean perch	0.4
Brook trout	0.4
Rock fish	0.3
Sturgeon	0.2
Yellowtail	0.2
Haddock	0.2
Yellow perch	0.2
Walleye	0.2
Atlantic cod	0.1
Northern pike	0.1
Sole	0.1

TABLE 13.3

BEST SOURCES OF OMEGA-3 ACIDS

Source	Gms, Omega-3/100 Calories
Fish oil capsules	2.86
Salmon, sockeye	1.71
Tuna, Albacore or longfin	1.22
Salmon, pink humpback	1.15
Shark: Spiny dogfish	1.14
Halibut: Atlantic	1.13
Anchovy	1.10
Salmon: Atlantic	1.08
Meckerel: Atlantic	1.08
Salmon: Pacific	1.03
Spanish sardne	0.91
Trout, rainbow, lake	0.86
Meckerel, Pacific	0.85
Swordfish, herring (pacific)	0.75

TABLE 13.4

WORST SOURCES OF OMEGA-3 ACIDS

Sole
Monkfish
Mackerel (except Atlantic/pacific)
Pike
Cod
Haddock
Pompano
Herring
Flounder
Buffalo or Sucker
Bass
Barracuda

Another consideration in the choice of fish is the quantity of cholesterol, especially in shellfish and oysters, which have been historically, but erroneously, considered rich in cholesterol (table 13.5).

TABLE 13.5

CHOLESTEROL CONTENT OF SELECTED FISH

Fish	Cholesterol, milligram/100 gram
Salmon	35
Tuna	38
Clams, softshell	25
Clams, hardshell	40
Swordfish	48
Oysters	50
Shrimp	66
Trout, brook	68
Lobster	70
Crab	76
Squid	250

Therefore, except for squid, all fish and shellfish are low in cholesterol compared to other meats. The U.S. Department of Health and Human Services and the Department of Agriculture currently recommend as many as four fish meals a week; the average American eats only one. Several recent studies have shown that even two fish meals a week can have a substantial beneficial effect.

Comparing the fish the Eskimos eat and the fish we eat, is not entirely fair, however. The fish consumed by Japanese fisherman and Eskimos is eaten raw, or only slightly cooked by steam or smoked, whereas we broil, charbroil, fry, bake, poach, bread, or cajun fish before eating it. The cooking process or the trimmings which come with fish can interfere with the absorption of the components of fish.

When fish is cooked with shortening (table 5.3), either vegetable or animal, frequent use of fish will cause the body to accumulate omega-6 or saturated fats. For example, a 3-oz serving of breaded fish has about 15 grams of fat added to it because of the cooking method. Such additions of fat to the diet defeat the purpose of a fish diet since the beneficial effects of omega-3 fatty acids are related to the ratio of omega-3 to omega-6 acids in the blood and not on the quantity of omega-3 acids alone. This is because the two types of acids compete for enzymes in the blood to produce the PGs. If both types of acids are taken in large quantity, the ratio will remain unchanged in the blood, a situation which can be potentially more harmful than when no fish is taken.

The Eskimos have an added advantage in that the raw fat they consume does not get exposed to air and is, therefore, less rancid and less likely to cause blocked arteries and cancer.

Also, the loss of vitamin A and other antioxidants during cooking renders our fish diet less effective in protecting from cancer. Does that mean, we should raw fish? Not at all; raw fish can cause infections that affect the brain. (Note: Eskimos show substantially higher incidence of psychotic disorder. Could there be a connection with eating raw meat?) Fish should be cooked in a manner which preserves its nutrition and

improves taste, yet eliminates the hazardous components. The best method of fish preparation is the moist-
heat technique such as poaching or steaming, which
adds few calories or carcinogens from burning, and
helps retain essential vitamins and minerals. The most
popular methods of fish preparation such as open fire
broiling (such as mesquite or blackened fish) and frying
are the worst when it comes to preserving the essential
qualities of a fish meal.

A recent study measured the omega-3 content of
an assortment of food served at fast-food chains, including fried fishwiches, fried chicken, hamburgers and
pepperoni pizza. All of these products had very low
omega-3 content with pizza topping the list. It is suspected that omega-3 acids can be destroyed when food
is fried. If one lesson can be learned from this study,
it is to avoid fast-food fish sandwiches, which may be
foisted upon us as the popularity of fish increases in
this country. The fast-food fish sandwich is higher in fat
than either a four-ounce hamburger or a white meat
chicken entree. The fast food fish sandwich is nearly
one-third lower in protein than either hamburger or chick-
en; breading and frying adds additional calories and
cholesterol to fish topping a quarter-pound hamburger.

While scientists explore the effects of cooking on
fish, and until the results are in, it is more logical to
consume fish oil capsules (4-10 perday) while continu-
ing to increase the use of fish (twice a week) to supply
the needed omega-3 acids in the body. In either event,
you must also take supplements of vitamin E, whose
absorption is reduced by omega-3 fatty acids.

In the following paragraphs we will discuss the advantages of fish oil and then follow up with Tables 13.6 and 13.7, listing the disadvantages of each. Most fish oils contain about equal quantities of saturated and polyunsaurated fats. However, fish oils can be made more unsaturated by a process called de-waxing, where the fatty acids are separated based on their freezing points. If you are taking fish oil supplements, put a few capsules in your freezer. You will find that about half of the oil in the capsule turns cloudy. This is the saturated, or less unsaturated, fraction of the oil. Better processing of oils in the future is expected to reduce their saturated fat content.

Each soft-gelatin capsule of fish oil has about 10 calories and, considering the recommended daily dose, it supplies about 40 to 60 calories compared to about 80 to 250 calories, in a typical 4-ounce fish serving, excluding the trimmings and the calories added due to the cooking process. If you eat fish and take fish oil supplements regularly, you must watch your total caloric intake. You may want to combine low calorie fish (less than 100 calories per meal) such as cod, haddock, perch, pike, rockfish or sole, with fish oil supplements to reduce total calories. Remember, however, that fish low in fat and calories are also low in omega-3 content.

The cholesterol content in fish oil supplements is about 5 milligrams/gram, approximately 10 times higher than in fish. However, the quantity of fish oil consumed, such as 4-6 grams per day gives only about one-half of the cholesterol found in an average seafood meal.

To a purist, who suspects, perhaps rightfully so, that there may be more than just omega-3 acids giving fish its magic healing ability, eating fish is the only way to good health. To a pragmatist, eating fish daily is no fun and he suspects that the fish we buy at the grocery store may contain many undesirable components as well.

A negative consideration in the use of fish is the pollution of marine and fresh waters with heavy metals, pesticides and other industrial chemicals such as PCB (polychlorinated biphenyls) which is banned from production, yet still exists in the environment. The fresh water fish is more likely to be contaminated chemically than the deep sea variety. The maximal allowed tolerance of PCB in fish is only 2 ppm (parts per million), yet even that amount can be harmful to pregnant and nursing women. Fortunately, PCB contamination is decreasing and you need not be concerned about it or other contaminants unless you eat a lot of fish caught in the polluted waters of the Great Lakes. Recently some of the Great Lakes have been cleaned and may not pose a threat as great as they did some years ago. Rainbow trout raised commercially or fished from clear mountain streams generally are safer.

When making a choice, you should also keep in mind that as a matter of convenience and consistency in dosing, many medical investigations have used fish oil supplements in place of fish diet to study the effect of omega-3 acids on the body. Many scientists who are involved in doing research on omega-3 fatty acids themselves take these capsules along with fish.

It is best to start slowly to determine tolerance to such a regimen. Start by taking two capsules per day, one with each meal during the first week. If no discomfort is felt, you can increase the dose to four to six capsules per day, taken over the course of the day but always with a meal, to assure maximum absorption (food in the stomach causes release of intestinal juices which help absorption of oils). Taking fish oil capsules on an empty stomach may cause local discomfort.

As expected, the purists and the fish industry are heavily promoting the use of fish, whereas the fish oil industry, an offshoot of natural health food industry and the soft gelatin capsule manufacturers, is pushing the use of fish oil supplements to keep our arteries supple and and hearts beating.

The debate has heated up during the past few months as several natural health food suppliers have started promoting fish oil. Many noted scientists are totally opposed to the idea of using fish oil supplements. An equal number of scientists would not leave home without their golden pills. Based on information in this book, you should be able to decide for yourself.

TABLE 13.6

DISADVANTAGES OF EATING FISH

Allergic reactions: due to fish proteins.

Microbiologic contamination: raw shellfish can cause hepatitis or food poisoning.

Chemical contamination: Many carcinogenic chemicals and pesticides are frequently found in lake fish.

Carcinogenesis: due to rotten fish (free radicals). Heavy metal poisoning: mercury, iron, copper, zinc or selenium, specially in crustaceous fish or mollusks.

Vitamin overdosing: vitamin A & D.

Monounsaturated fatty acids: gadoleic and cetoleic acids in fish can make heart "fatty"; several other undesirable fatty acids also exist in fish.

Variable quantity of omega-3 acids: fish processing, preservation.

Loss of omega-3 acids during cooking: the vitamin loss during cooking ranges from 10-50%.

TABLE 13.7

DISADVANTAGES OF TAKING FISH OIL SUPPLEMENTS

Missing other essential components.

Incomplete absorption: especially in diseases of fat malabsorption.

Local effects: stomach or intestine irritation or allergic response possible.

Regurgitation: after taste.

Vitamin absorption: reduces absorption of fat soluble vitamins such as E.

Chemical contamination: possibly in a more concentrated form; also, contaminants from the process of manufacturing.

Prolonged bleeding times: interaction for patients on anticoagulant therapy; possible problems in surgery and injuries.

Excessive caloric intake: equivalent calories to other oils; 10 g/day is 36,000 calories per year.

The world currently produces about 2.5 billion pounds of crude fish oil; the U.S. production of 250 million pounds is primarily exported since the government regulations will not allow it to be used here. The U.S. market alone should hover around one billion pounds of crude oil per year, allowing about 5 grams of oil per day for each citizen. Considering the current retail cost of about 5 cents per one gram capsule, this represents a $24 billion market in the U.S. and a half a trillion dollar market worldwide. The U.S. stands an excellent chance of becoming the world's largest exporter of oil, a crude of a different kind.

Fish Oil Components

The beneficial components of fish oil, particularly EPA and DHA, are being studied by major pharmaceutical companies for possible use as drugs in the treatment of the various ailments already discussed. Also, these acids are now prepared in an ester form (a chemically modified form), which is purported to be better absorbed and tolerated. It won't be very long until we see EPA and DHA fortified products appearing on the market. However, the arguments presented against the use of fish oil over fish are also applicable here: the EPA and DHA alone may not be as effective as the complete oil, whose additional components may either improve the effectiveness of EPA and DHA or provide unique actions of their own.

Most of the commercial fish oils contain 180 milligram of EPA and 120 milligram of DHA per gram of oil. Since EPA is more important than DHA in modfiying eicosanoids in the body, the best fish oils have highest concentration of EPA (table 13.8). The total quantity of EPA and DHA in a fish meal also depends on the percentage of fat.

TABLE 13.8

EPA & DHA CONTENT(%) OF FISH OILS

OIL	EPA	DHA
Atlantic manheden	17	7
S. African mackarel	16	12
Japanese sardine	16	11
Red fish	12	15
Cod	11	21
Iceland capelin	9	11
Flounder	9	9
Atlantic herring	9	6
Albacore tuna	9	25
Chinook salmon	8	5
Iceland cod liver	8	9
Canadian tuna	7	20
Pacific halibut	6	10
Michigan salmon	3	6
Mexican anchovy	1	32
Mississippi catfish	0.5	0.5

Notice that fish like Mexican anchovy are extremely high in total omega-3 concentration but have very little EPA. Salmon has generally high quantities of omega-3 fatty acids because of its fatty nature, even though the concentration of acids is low. Fish high in DHA may be recommended for children who need larger supply of DHA.

DO WE REALLY NEED EITHER?

There are alternate sources of omega-3 acids available abundantly in nature. Various omega-3-rich marine plants such as chlorella (sp. minutissime) or plankton are good sources, which can be a substitute for fish oil. These marine vegetables, along with the more common ones we know, can be processed directly into foods, ala tofu, at a much cheaper cost than extracting oil from fish. Linseed, soybean and rapseed oil also provide omega-3 fatty acids but these are of the type which is not as effective as the omega-3 fatty acids found in fish (table 13.9). It should be remembered that fish is merely a storage medium for omega-3 acids; it can not produce these acids. For example, cultured catfish raised on soybean meal has very little EPA or DHA.

The fish derive their supply of omega-3 acids from marine plants; smaller fish are eaten by larger fish, which are in turn eaten by even larger fish or mammals like whales, whose blubbers end up on the dinner table in remote igloos some 300 miles north of the polar circle on Greenland's barren west coast. And that's how Eskimos benefit from the vegetables in the sea. Do we have to go this long route to obtain our supply of omega-3 acids? Not necessarily. We can go straight to the source of omega-3 acids (table 13.9) and cut out all the fish in between. But, would eating algae be as much fun as a steamed salmon? Quite possibly. Ask a salmon.

TABLE 13.9

SOURCES OF OMEGA-3 FATTY ACIDS

Source	% Omega-3	(EPA + DHA)	% Omega-6
Fish Oils	13-35	27-30	1-14
Land Plant Oils			
Linseed	26-58	0	5-23
Soybean	2-10	0	49-52
Rapseed	1-10	0	10-22

Marine Plants			
Seaweeds	50-60	15-25	3-10
Phytoplankters	12-39	10-32	1-2
Copepod	20-24	20-21	1-2

The vegetable source of omega-3 acids are quite limited. Also, the type of omega-3 acids found in terrestrial plants are of less benefit to health (EPA and DHA are best for health). However, marine plants have great abundance of omega-3 acids. Can we harvest them? Most definitely. There are also unlimited possibilities with genetic engineering of plants to produce omega-3 fatty acids.

Is it possible that we may have overlooked other sources of omega-3 acids in plants which are not generally part of our food? There is a need to examine plants which grow in colder and moist climates for their omega-3 content. In the meantime, the seabed is full of heart-comforting weeds and we no longer need to feel gulty about cultivating weeds.

The chemical synthesis of omega-3 fatty acids is likely to yield highly purified forms of these acids in sufficient quantity to supply the entire world. However, any significant increase in our omega-3 intake would come only if our routine diets are made abundant in omega-3 fatty acids. One way to accomplish this would be to fortify the cattle and poultry feeds with omega-3 acids. This will allow beef and chicken meat to serve the same purpose as does the blubber for the Eskimos. Beef, because of its fatty nature, would be an ideal source to store omega-3 acids.

Health Foods

The race is on. It should not come as a surprise to anyone to see a plethora of health foods containing fish oil or its components hit the markets. And with that will come claims of ultimate superiority of one product over another. New formulations of fish oils will probably contain egg white, refined lecithin, soybean sterols, apple fiber, vitamin E, and garlic as additives to improve efficacy of the active ingredients. It will be interesting to see the imaginative products developed from fish oil in the future. Some recommendations include DHA fortified infant formula, deodorized cooking oils derived from fish or sea vegetation, EPA and DHA based artificial milk, meal replacement plans based on marine algae, etc.

14
THE FDA

*"It ain't no sin if you
crack a few laws now and then,
just so long as you don't break any."*

**MAE WEST, in
Every Day's a Holiday(1937).**

The distribution of drugs and foods is governed
in this country by an agency of the U.S. government,
The Food and Drug Administration (FDA). By defini-
tion, any product carrying claims to prevent or treat
any body condition is a drug. And no drug can be sold
in the U.S. without prior approval by the FDA, a process
which takes several years and millions of dollars to
satisfy the FDA study guidelines. As a result, the well-
heeled drug industry only pursues those drugs which
are either patented or have proprietary protection to
allow them to recoup their investment in seeking FDA
approval. A large number of very effective drugs, therefore, never reach consumers.

In view of the fast-breaking news regarding the

applications of fish oils, recommendation to use them to treat an ailment or prevent it, will throw this food product into the drug classification as defined by the FDA. It is unlikely that any drug company will undertake studies under the FDA guidelines to seek approval of therapeutic claims since there is no proprietary protection on the product. However, the evidence regarding the beneficial effects of fish oils is mounting every day and the FDA may be forced to allow label claims of some sort such as happened in the case of Kellogg's All Bran Cereal, which is permitted to carry a claim that it can prevent cancer because of its high fiber content.

Some drug companies are already testing the waters by openly advertising in the print media and through television that their products help reduce heart disease, cancer, migraine, etc. This must be quite frustrating for the FDA. Can they force such promotional campaigns to be withdrawn? Yes. But are they going to do it? That will depend on the opinion of the public and the scientific community.

Many highly reputable and influential scientists still do not believe that fish oil supplements have any therapeutic value. It is ironic that such overwhelming evidence can be overlooked. It's too bad fish does not cure myopic vision. However, an informed public is soon going to learn what fish oils are all about, which will make it almost impossible for the FDA to whip this product.

In the meantime, until the FDA allows it to be sold as a drug, fish oil will continue selling as food with such guarded claims as: "to help reduce the risk of heart disease" and "as part of a total dietary plan to reduce overall fat consumption and increase the ratio of polyunsaturated to saturated fats—an increased intake of fish rich in omega-3 polyunsaturates can help lower plasma lipid levels and reduce the risk of atherosclerotic disease."

This "cat and mouse" game between the FDA and the fish oil manufacturers must end in the best interest of the public health. The FDA must take a definite position on this product. If you call the FDA (1-202-485-0233), they will tell you that any fish oil product with direct or implied claim for any effect on the body is "misbranded" and illegal for sale in this country. It is, however, perfectly legal to sell and buy fish oil without these therapeutic claims. Yet, if you visit your local supermarket, you will find many products on the shelves, in clear violation of these regulations. Is the FDA doing its job? Yes and No. The FDA is currently in a wait and see posture. One possible solution to this problem may be to classify fish oil as "therapeutic food," like the GRAS List (generally regarded as safe) for chemicals which have been in use for long time and have been proven safe anecdotally. But there remain many regulatory snafus; for example, in this country, a great deal of fish oil is produced from Atlantic menhaden— some 100,000 tons. However, it cannot be sold as a food because it is not on the GRAS list. So the menhaden oil is exported to Europe, where it is partially hydrogenated to vegetable oil or margarine-like consistency.

This is not, however, the first time that the FDA finds itself in such a dilemma. In the past, for example, as a result of public outcry and congressional pressure,

the FDA studied the anti-cancer properties of grapefruit
pits (laetrile) and found them to be ineffective. Doesn't
fish oil deserve at least as much respect as the grapefruit
pits? Write to the FDA and your congressman about it.

15

THE ULTIMATE PANACEA

*"I firmly believe that if
the whole MATERIA MEDICA could
be sunk to the bottom of the sea,
it would be all the better for mankind
and all the worse for the fishes."*

**O. W. Holmes,
LECTURE, Harvard Medical School**

Fish do not need the Materia Medica (a book describing sources and properties of drugs). They are the Materia Medica. Man has always been searching for a panacea for his ailments. He has just found one in the deep seas. Fish itself has no curative properties, it merely undoes what our diets do to us. Fish fat provides the missing link necessary to maintain the delicate balance of the effects of our diets on our body. It would seem ruthless, if nature had not provided, equally abundantly, the antidotes to its own deleterious offerings in the form of delicious fats.

Given the passion Americans have for fatty foods, it is unlikely that any serious dent will be made in the total fat consumption within the next century and consequently damage to our arteries, brain, and the rest of the body will continue. However, supplementing our diets with fish or fish oils offers a prophylaxis against our diets. Finally, for dessert lovers, there is hope.

Far from being an ordinary "fish story," this book has been the extraordinary account of one of the exciting medical discoveries of the century. It was written in the hope that through education, the consumer will grasp the chance to preserve health and increase his lifespan through the use of fish.

16

APPENDIX

APPENDIX A-1

FATTY ACIDS AND THEIR SOURCES

Fatty Acid	#Cs	Common Source
SATURATED:		
Acetic	2	Vinegar, carbohydrate fermentation
Butyric	4	Butter
Caproic	6	Butter
Caprylic	8	Butter, other plant fats
Decanoic	10	Butter, other plant fats
Lauric	12	Cinnamon, palm kernel, coconut oil, laurels
Myristic	14	Nutmeg, palm kernel, coconut oil, mystels, all animal and fish fat
Palmitic	16	All animal and plant fats
Stearic	18	All animal and plant fats
Arachidic	20	Peanut (arachis oil)
Lignoceric	24	Peanut

UNSATURATED: (Unsaturation site/omega position)		
Oleic	18(1/9)	All fats
Linoleic	18(2/6)	Corn, peanut/cotton seed/soybean
Linolenic	18(3/3)	Above plus linseed oil
Arachidonic	18(4/6)	Mainly peanut oil
Eicosapentaenoic	18(5/3)	Fish, marine plants
Docosahexaenoic	22(6/3)	Fish, marine plants

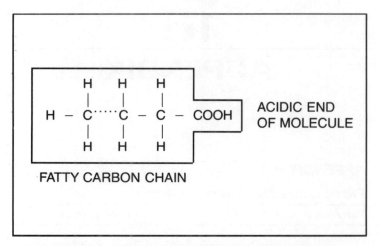

APPENDIX A-2 **Saturated fatty acid structure**

H – C#–C – C = C – C – COOH

    1   2   3   4   5 = No. of C atom

\# = Terminal or OMEGA carbon
* = missing hydrogen atoms

APPENDIX A-3 **Unsaturated omega fatty acid structure**

APPENDIX A-4

CLASSIFICATION/COMPOSITION OF LIPOPROTEINS

Density Lipids	(%) Protein	TRIG	PHLPD	CHL	FFA
Ultra low	-4	1	87	8	40	
Very low	-4 to 0	7	53	18	21	1
Low	0 to 6	16	18	23	42	1
High	6 to 21	45	8	25	20	2
Very High	over 28	99	0	0	0	1

KEY—TRIG: triglycerides; PHLPD: phospholipids; CH: cholesterol; FFA: free fatty acids; %: percentage heavier compared to water.

APPENDIX A-5

SPECIFIC ACTIVITIES OF EICOSANOIDS*

Prostaglandin E_2 (PGE$_2$)	Dilates vessels, inhibits stomach acids, promotes cancers
Thromboxane A_2 (THX$_2$)	Causes clotting of platelets
Thromboxane A_3 (THX$_3$)	Inactive
Prostacycline (PGI$_2$)	Dilates vessels, prevents clots
Prostacycline (PGI$_3$)	Dilates vessels, prevents clots
Leukotriene B_4 (LTB$_4$)	Promotes defense mechanism
HETE A_5	Promotes defense mechanism

* The subscript indicates the number of unsaturation sites; the series-2 PGs are produced by omega-6 fatty acids derived from vegetable oils and the series-3 PGs are derived mainly from fish fatty acids. Thromboxane and prostacycline are the types of PGs.

APPENDIX A-6 Role of fatty acid in plaque formation

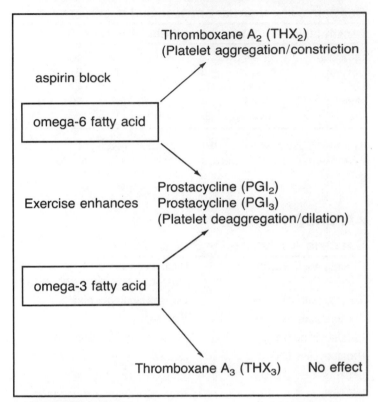

APPENDIX A-7
DIETARY FAT IN ESKIMO AND DANISH FOODS

Dietary Fat	Eskimos	Danes
Energy (3,000 cal)	39%	42%
Saturated fat	23%	53%
Monounsaturated	58%	34%
Polyunsaturated	19%	13%
omega-3 fat	14%	3%
omega-6 fat	5%	10%
Cholesterol	0.79 g/day	0.42 g/day
P/S ratio	0.84	0.24

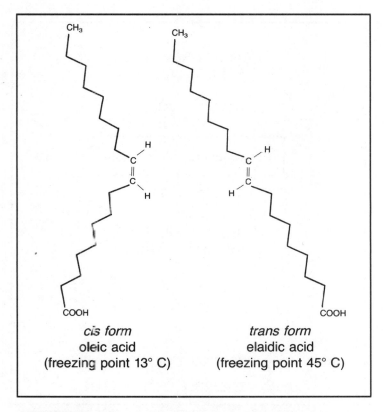

cis form
oleic acid
(freezing point 13° C)

trans form
elaidic acid
(freezing point 45° C)

APPENDIX A-8 **Unnatural fatty acids in margarine.**
*(The unnatural trans form has a much higher freezing point and helps
keep margarine solid at room temperature.)*

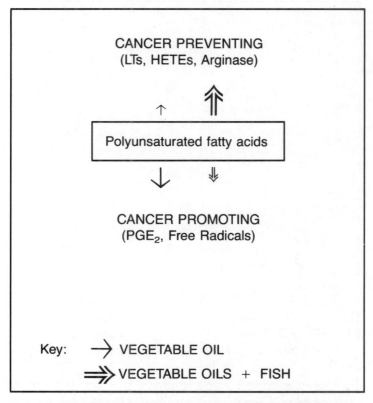

APPENDIX A-9   HOW FISH PREVENT CANCER

APPENDIX A-10

CHARACTERISTICS OF FISH FATTY ACIDS

Acid Freezing	°C	#US*	Omega	Source
Myristic	55	0	n/a	all animal and fish
Decenoic	145	1	1	sperm head, butter, milk
Lauroleic	?	1	7	sperm blubber, head oil
Physeteric	?	1	9	whale blubber, sardines
Palmitoleic	1	1	7	marine oils, fat depot
Gadoleic	25	1	11	marine oils, veg. oils
Eicosenoic	22	1	9	fish oils, mustard, jojoba
Cetoleic	33	1	11	marine oils
Stelacholeic	41	1	9	shark and ray liver oils
Hiragonic	?	3	2	sardine oils
Stearadonic	?	4	?	marine oils
Timnodonic	-60	5	2	sardine, cod liver, whale
Eicosapentaenoic	-80	5	3	fish oils, about 12%
Docosahexaenoi	-84	6	3	fish oils, about 18%
Clupanodonic	-78	5	3	fish oils, small qty

* # of unsaturation sites.

17

GLOSSARY

Allergy

Defensive responsive of the body to "foreign elements." Includes symptoms of cold, asthma, etc.

Aneurism

Distension of blood vessels; may cause rupture or leakage of blood.

Antioxidants

Chemicals which combines with oxygen and free radicals to prevent fats and oils from becoming oxidized or rancid. Examples include vitamins A, C, E, B-1, B-5, B-6, the amino acid cysteine, the food antioxidants BHA (butylated hydroxyanisole) and BHT (butylated hydroxytoluene) and minerals such as selenium and zinc. Antioxidants help prevent cancer and heart disease.

Arachidonic Acid

An unsaturated, 20-carbon long, omega-6 fatty acid, the principal precursor to eicosanoids (such as prostaglandins) which cause narrowing of blood vessels and blood clotting. Found in vegetable oils, mainly peanut oil. Several fatty acids in the body convert to arachidonic acid.

Arginase

Enzyme which enhances the infection-fighting ability of the body's defense system (macrophages).

Arteriosclerosis

Diseases characterized by thickening and loss of the elasticity of arterial walls, comprising three distinct forms: atherosclerosis, Monckeberg's arteriosclerosis and arteriolosclerosis.

Atherocyte (Atheroma)

A mass or plaque of degenerated, thickened arterial lining occurring in atherosclerosis.

Atherosclerosis

An extremely common form of arteriosclerosis in which deposits of yellowish plaque (atheromas) containing cholesterol and other lipids are formed within the wall of the arteries, mainly that of heart, brain and legs causing heart attacks, angina pains, strokes, and poor blood circulation.

Carcinogens

Cancer producing substances such as a chemicals, ultraviolet radiation, free radicals, or viruses.

Carcinoma

Cancerous tissue growth.

Cardiovascular system

Pertaining to heart and blood vessels.

Cell wall

The outer structure of the cell.

Coronary artery

The blood vessels supplying blood to heart.

Cyclooxygenase

The enzyme required for the conversion of fatty acids, such as arachidonic acid. to eicosanoids. Many anti-inflammatory drugs, such as aspirin, act by inactivating this enzyme. Omega-3 fatty acids react with cyclooxygenase enzyme to produce less harmful eicosanoids.

Docosahexaenoic acid (DHA)

An unsaturated, 22-carbon long, omega-3 fatty acid found mainly in fish and marine plants. Most commercial fish oil preparations contain 12 percent DHA. Considered important for brain and eye development, especially in children.

Eicosanoids

Hormone-like substances formed mainly by arachidonic acid, an omega-6 acid; two main types of eicosanoids are prostaglandins and leukotrienes. Eicosanoids control blood pressure, blood clotting, body's infection fighting ability, allergic responses, etc.

Eicosapentaenoic acid (EPA)

An unsaturated, 20-carbon long, omega-3 fatty acid found in fish and marine plants. Most commercial fish oil preparations contain 18 percent EPA. Considered as the major reason for the beneficial effects of fish oils. Acts by producing eicosanoids which are beneficial to the body.

Essential Fatty Acids

The fatty acids that the body cannot synthesize but needs for normal metabolism. These include linoleic acid, linolenic acid, and arachidonic acid. Also termed as vitamin F. Deficiency of essential fatty acids, a rare occurrence, causes skin diseases.

Fatty Acids

Long chain carbon acidic compounds found frequently in nature, they could be saturated or unsaturated. They also act as a precursor to various eicosanoids.

FDA

The Food and Drug Administration, a regulatory authority of the U.S. government which approves and regulates the distribution of drugs and foods.

Free radicals

Highly activated and charged forms of molecules which interact rapidly with body tissues causing cancer and atherosclerosis.

High density lipids (HDL or VHDL)

Mixture of triglycerides, cholesterol and other fats and proteins. Generally considered to be beneficial to heart. Heavier than water, by 6 to 28 percent.

Hydroxyeicosatetraenoic acid (HETE)

An eicosanoid which controls many body functions including the body immune defense system.

Hypertension

High blood pressure.

Immune response

Defensive response of body to "foreign elements."

Inflammation

A localized protective response to destroy, or dilute or wall off (sequester) both the injurious agent and the injured tissue. Examples include arthritis, swelling upon injuries, etc.

Inuits

People who eat raw fish, refers to Eskimos.

Low density lipids (LDL)

Mixtures of triglycerides, cholesterol and other fats and proteins (less than HDL). Generally considered extremely dangerous to heart. Weigh less than water.

Lipids

Chemicals which are insoluble in water but soluble in alcohol, ether and chloroform and other fat solvents and which have a greasy feel. These include fatty acids, neutral fats, waxes, cholesterol, steroids and phosphatides.

Lipoproteins

Combined forms of lipids and proteins; makes lipids more water soluble and dispersible in blood.

Lipooxygenase

The enzyme responsible for converting fatty acids to eicosanoids such as HETEs and LTs.

Leukotrienes (LT)

Eicosanoids which control many body systems such

as the body's defense mechanism.

Macrophage

Any large cell with the ability to engulf other cells, generally found in the walls of the blood vessels. They are usually immobile but when stimulated by inflammation they become actively mobile and move throughout the body.

Marine Lipid Concentrate

Fish oil obtained from fish generally by a cold process of squeezing the fish. Most commercial preparations contain 18 percent EPA and 12 percent DHA.

Omega-3

Refers to the third carbon in the fatty acid molecule which is unsaturated, counting from the carbon terminal end. Omega-3 fatty acids are found in fish, marine plants, and some terrestrial plants.

Omega-6

Refers to the sixth carbon in the fatty acid molecule which the unsaturated, counting from the carbon terminal end. Omega-6 are found mainly in vegetable oils.

Oxidation

Addition of oxygen to a chemical structure. In oils, oxidation causes rancidity, which is a possible cause for the carcinogenesis of oils.

Polyunsaturated

Fatty acids with more than one unsaturated carbon.

Polyunsaturated oils freeze at lower temperatures than the monounsaturated and saturated oils and fats and are preferred to reduce risk of heart disease.

Prostacyclines (PGI)

A type of prostaglandins (PGs) produced by the lining of the artery; decrease blood clotting and expand blood vessels resulting in reduced plaque formation and blood pressure.

Prostaglandins (PGs)

Eicosanoids produced from arachidonic acid. PGs stimulate contraction of uterus and other muscles, lower blood pressure and assist in the action of certain hormones. First found in semen, they have been found in arterial lining, menstrual fluid and other body tissues.

Saturated Fatty Acids

Fatty acids with saturated structure. Found in all fats, particularly animal fats. Highly dangerous to body health, causing atherosclerosis.

Steroids

Lipid of high molecular weight, serve as precursor for various vitamins and hormones. Examples include vitamin D, cholesterol, etc.

Thromboxane (THX)

A type of eicosanoid which causes clotting of blood and increases stickiness of platelets. The thromboxane produced from omega-3 fatty acids is devoid of any activity.

Triglycerides

Common fat. Made up of three molecules of fatty acid and one molecule of glycerol. Part of all blood lipids, especially, the low density types, which are particularly harmful to the body.

Ultra low density lipids (ULDL)

Also called chylomicrons. Very large in size and of fluffy characteristics.

Very high density lipids (VHDL)

Consist mainly of proteins and fatty acids.

Very low density lipids (VLDL)

Much lighter-than-water fraction of blood lipids, highly dangerous to health.

18

BIBLIOGRAPHY

1987:

Neal, Charles, D. (1987). A fish story. *Prevention* 39:14

1986:

Altschyle, M. D. (1986). A tale of two lipids. Cholesterol and eicosapentaenoic acid. *Chest* 35(5):601-602.

Aursnes, I. Dorum, H. P. Smith, P. Arnesen, H. Christiansen, E. N. Norum, K. R. Fischer, S. Weber, P. C. (1986). Low and high risk coronary patients discriminated by blood platelet fatty acid composition. *Scand. J. Clin. Lab. Invest.* 46(2):115-120.

Aviram, M. Brox, J. Nordoy, A. (1986). Acute effects of dietary cod liver oil and cream on plasma lipoproteins. *Ann. Nutr. Metab.* 30(2):143-148.

Casalio, R. E., et al. (1986). Improved graft patency associated with altered platered functions induced by marine fatty acids in dogs. *Thrombosis Haemostasis* 50(4):762-67.

Davidson, M. (1936). Marine lipid concentrate reduces coronary risk factors, Double-blind comparison with olive oil (abstract). *J. Am. Coll. Cardiol.* 7(Suppl A): 247A.

Davidson, M. Lieoson, P. R. (1986). Marine lipids and Atherosclerosis. *Cardiovasc. Rev. Rep.* 7(5):461-472.

Dushcek, Jeanie. (1986). Fish, fatty acids, and physiology; Fish, long called brain food, turns out to be heart food as well. *Science News* October 19:1986, 252(3)

Dyberg, J. (1986). Linoleate-derived polyunsaturated fatty acids and prevention of atherosclerosis. *Nutr. Rev.* 44(4):125-134.

Gutierrez, Vallejo, F. Gutierrez, Rosch, F. Guiterrez, Rosch, R. Rodriguez, Fernandez, R. Ortiz, Errano A. (1986). Effects of cod liver oil on lipids, lipoproteins and platelet function in patients with atherosclerotic vasculopathy. 1. Atheroscleros s therapy, basic concepts. 2. Clinical study, Conclusions. *Angiologia* 38(1): 7-31.

Hadjiagapio C., et al. (1986). Eicosapentaenoic acid utilization by Bovine aortic endothelial cells, effects on prostacyclin production. *Biochim. Biophys. Acta* 875(2):369-381.

Herold, P. M. Kinsella, J. E. (1986). Fish oil comsumption and decreased risk of cardiovascular disease, a comparison of findings from animal and human feeding trials. *Am. J. Clin. Nutr.* 43(4):566-598.

Illman, R. J., Trimble, R. P., Storer, G. B., Oliver, J. R. (1986). Time course changes in plasma lipids in diabetic rats fed diets high in fish or safflower oils. *Atherosclerosis* 59(3):313-321.

Kahn, A., Jr. (1986). Fish—more than a past-time [Editorial]. *J. Arkansas Med. Soc.* 82(8):392-393.

Kamada, T. Yamashita, T. Baba, Y. Kai, M. Setoyama, S. Chuman, Y. Otsuji, S. (1986). Dietary sardine oil increases erythrocyte membrane fluidity in diabetic patients. *Diabetes* 35(5):604-611.

Kelley, V. E. Sneve, S. Musinski, S. (1986). Increased renal thromboxane production in murine lupus nephritis. *J. Clin. Invest.* 77(1):252-259.

Knapp, H. R. Reilly, I. A. Alessandrini, P. Fitzgerald, G. A. (1986). In vivo indexes of platelet and vascular
function during fish-oil administration in patients with atherosclerosis. *N. Engl. J. Med.* 314(15): 937-942.

Lands, William, E. M. (1986). Renewed questions about polyunsaturated fatty acids. *Nutr. Rev.* 44(6):189-195.

Landymore. R. W. Macaulay, M. Sheridan, B. Cameron, C. (1986). Comparison of cod-liver oil and aspirin-dipyridamole for the prevention of intimal hyperplasia in autologuous vein grafts. *Ann. Thorac. Surg.* 41(1):54-57.

Leaf, Alexander. (1986). Fish Story. (Fish oil reduces chances of atherosclerosis). *Harvard Medical School Health Letter* 5:3.

Lee, T. H. Arm, J. P. (1986). Prospects for modifying the allergic response by fish oil diets. *Clin. Allergy* 16(2):89-100.

Lee, T. H. Isreal, E. Drazen, J. M. Leitch, A, G. Ravalese, J., III. Corey, E. J. Robinson, D. R. Lewis, R. A. Austen, K. (1986). Enhancement of plasma levels of biologically active leukotriene B compounds during anaphylaxis in guinea pigs pretreated by indomethacin or by a fish oil-enriched diet. *J. Immunol.* 136(7):2575-2582.

Meade, Jeff. (1986). Nutritional breakthrough of the 80's, Omega-3. *Prevention* 38:85-88.

Nestel, P. J. (1986). Fish Oil attenuates the cholesterol induced rise in lipoprotein cholesterol. *Am. J. Clin. Nutr.* 43(5):752-757.

Neuringer, Martha, and Connor, William, E. (1986). n-3 fatty acids in the brain and retina, Evidence for their essentiality. *Nutr. Rev.* 44(9):285-294.

Norris, P. G., et al. (1986). Effect of dietary supplementation with fish oil on systolic blood pressure in mild essential hypertension. *Br. Med. J.* 293:104-105.

Norell, E. L. et al. (1986). Fish consumption and mortality from coronary heart disease. *Br. Med. J.* 293:426.

Robinson, D. R. Prickett, J. D. Makul G. T. Steinberg, A. D. Colvin, R. B. (1986). Dietary fish oil reduces progression of established renal disease in (NZB x NZW). F1 mice and delays renal disease in BXSB and MRL/1 strains *Arthritis-Rheum.* 29(4):539-546.

Rovner, Sandy (1986). Fish oil's new fame, It may have a positive role to play in the diet. How big is yet to be determined. *Washington Post* 109(Wed):16, Col. 4

Singer, P. Virth, M. Mest, H. J. Taube, C. Richter, Heinrich, E. Godicke, W. Hartrodt, W. Naumann, E. Voigt, S. (1986). Changes in blood pressure and serum lipids with fish diets in patients with mild essential hyper-tension. *Z. Gesante. Inn. Med.* 41(2):38-44.

Siwolop, Sana (1986). A fish a day may keep the paramedic away. (Fish oil beleived to prevent hardening of the arteries). *Business Week* May 26:85.

Sugiyama, H. Sand, M. (1986). Health food containing unsaturated fatty acid residue-glyceride and protein. *Jpn. Kokai. Tokyo Koho.* JP 61(15):649.

Thorngren, A. Nilsson, E. Gustafson, A. (1986). Plasma lipoproteins and fatty acid consumption during a moderate eicosapentaeonic acid diet. *Acta. Med. Scand.* 219(1):23-28.

Zamula, Evelyn. (1986). The Greenland diet, Can fish oils prevent heart disease? *FDA Consumer* 20(8):6-8.

No Author. 1986). Biochemical effects of marine fish oils in human subjects. *Nutr. Rev.* 44(6):205-207.

No Author. (1986). Fish and olive oils, Heart-healthy fare? (Lowering cholesterol). (Column. *Changing Times* 40:12(1).

No Author. (1986). Cod-liver oil may benefit patients with coronary artery disease. *Am. Fam. Physician* 33(2):265-267.

No Author. (1985). Dietary fish oil alters leukotriene generation and neutrophil function. *Nutr. Rev.* 44(4):137-139.

No Author. (1986). Plasma lipoproteins and fatty acid composition during a moderate eicosapentaenoic acid diet. *Acta Med. Scand.* 219(1):23-28.

No Author. (1986). Treatment of combined hyperlipidemia with fish and vegetable oils. *Nutr. Rev.* 44(4):140-142.

No Author. (1986). Cholesterol metabolism and omega-3 polyenes in fish oils. *Nutr. Rev.* 44(4):147.

No Author. (1986). Comparison of cod-liver and aspirin-dipyridamole for the prevention of intimal hyperplasia in autologous vein grafts. *Ann. Thor. Surg.* 41(1):54-57.

1985:

Adam, O. (1985). Nutrition physiology studies with foramula diets, Metabolism of multiple unsaturated fatty acids and prostaglandin biosynthesis in the human. *Klin. Wochenschr.* 63(16):731-739.

Arntzenius, A. C., et al. (1985). Diet, lipoproteins, and the progression of coronary atherosclerosis—The Leiden Intervention Trial. *New. Eng. J. Med.* 312:617-624.

Barcelli, U. Glas, Greenwalt P. Pollak, V. E. (1985). Enhancing effect of dietary supplementation with omega-3 fatty acids on plasma fibrinolysis in normal subjects. *Thromb. Res.* 39(3):307-312.

Bates, C., et al. (1985). Plasma essential fatty acids in pure and mixed rate american Indians on and off a diet exceptionally rich in salmon. *Prostaglandin Leukotrienes Med.* 17(1):77-84.

Begin, M. E., et al. (1985). Selective killing of human cancer cells by polyunsaturated fatty acids. *Prostaglandins Leukotrienes Med.* 19(2):117-186.

Bishop, Jerry E. (1985). Eating fish reduces heart-attack risk, researchers assert; a daily dish is seen having a therapeutic effect for middle-aged males. *Wall Street Journal* May 9:16.

Blankenhorn, M., et al. (1985). Two new diet-heart studies. *New Eng. J. Med.* 312:851.

Boberg, M. Vessby, B. Croon, L. B. (1985). Fatty acid composition of platelets and of plasma lipid esters in relation to platelet function in patients with ischamic heart disease. *Atherosclerosis* 58(1-3):49-63.

Boggio, S. M. Hardy, R. W. Babbitt, J. K. (1985). The influence of dietary lipid source and alpha tocopherol acetate level on product quality of rainbow trout. *Aquaculture* 51(1):13-24.

·Booyens, J. Van Der Merwe, C. F. Katzeff, I. E. (1985). Chronic arachidonic acid eicosanoid imbalance, A common feature in coronary artery disease, hyperchlosterolemia, cancer and other important diseases. Significance of desaturase enzyme inhibition and of the arachidonic acid desaturase-independent pathway. *Med. Hypotheses* 18(1):53-60.

Braesalier, R. S., and Kim, Y. S. (1985). Diet and colon cancer. *New Eng. J. Med.* 313:1413-1414.

Cartwright, I. J. Pockley, A. G. Galloway, J. H. Greaves, M. Preston, F. E. (1985 . The effects of dietary omega-3 Polyunsaturated fatty acids on erythrocyte membrane phospholipids, erythrocyte deformabi i:y and blood viscosity in hea thy volunteers. *Athreosclerosis* 55(3):267-281

Curb, J. D. Reed, D. M. (1985). Fish consumption and mortality from coronary heart disease. *New Eng. J. Med.* 313(3):821.

Decarvalho S. (1985). Atherosclerosis. I. A leiomyproli erative disease of the arteries resulting from breakdown of the endothelial barrier to potent blood growth factors. II. Perspectives in anthroprophylaxis. *Angiology* 36(10):697-710.

Gabor, H. A. (1985). Fish consumption and mortality from coronary heart disease. *New Eng. J. Med.* 313(13):823.

Glomset, J. A. (1985). Fish, fatty acids, and human health [Editorial]. *N. Engl. J. Med.* 312(19):1253-1254.

Goldberg, A. C. Schonfeld, G. (1985). Effects of diet on lipoprotein metabolism. *Annu. Rev. Nutr.* 5:195-212.

Green, D. Barreres, L. Borensztajn, J. Kaplan, P. Reddy, M. N. Rovner, R. Simon, H. (1985). A double-blind, placebo-controlled trial of fish oil concentrate (MaxEPA). in stroke patients. *Stroke* 15(4):706-709.

Kelsey, Richard. (1985). Under my skin: Using vitamin A in a fish-oil base to clear up warts). *Health* 1, May:12(1).

Knapp, H. L., and Fitzgerald, G. A. (1985). Dietary eicosapentaenoic acid and human atherosclerosis., *Atherosclerosis* Rev. 13:127-143.

Kobayashi, Y. Fukuo, Y. Nakazawa, Y. Kato, H. Yoshi, H. Inaba, H. Berger, I. Naumann, E. Listing, J. Hartrody, W. Tuabe, C. (1985). Blood pressure and lipid lowering effect of mackerel and herring diet r patients with mild essential hypertension. *Atherosclerosis* 56(2):223-235.

Kromhout, D. Bosschieter, E. Coulander, C. (1985). The inverse relation between fish consumption and 20 year mortality from coronary heart disease. *N. Engl. J. Med.* 312:1205-1209.

Lands, W. E. M., et al. (1985). Relationship of thromboxane generation to the aggregation and platelets from humans, effects of EPA., *Prostaglandins* 30(5):819.

Landymore, R. W. Kinley, C. E. Cooper, M. D., et al. (1985). Cod liver oil in the prevention of intimal hyperplasia in autogenous vein grafts used for aterial bypass. *J. Thorac. Cardiovasc. Surg.* 89:351-357.

Lee, T. H. Hoover, R. L. Williams, J. D. Sperling, R. I. Ravalese, J. D. Spur, B. W. Robinson, D. R. Corey, E. J. Lewis, R. A. Austen, K. F. (1985).

Effect of dietary enrichment with eicosapentaenoic and docosahexaenoic acids on in vitro neutrophil and monocyte leukotriene generation and neutrophil function. *N. Engl. J. Med.* 312(19):1217-1224.

Lee, T.H. Austen, K. F. Leitch, G. Isreal, E. Robinson, D. R. Lewis, R. A. Corey, E. J. Drazen, J. M. (1985). The effects of a fish-oil enriched diet on pulmonary mechanics during anaphylaxis. *Am. Rev. Respir. Dis.* 132(6):1204-1209.

Leslie, C. A., Gonnerman, W. A., Ullman, M. D., Hayes, K.C., Franzblau, C. (1985). Dietary fish oil modulates macrophage fatty acids and decreases arthritis susceptibility in mice. *J. Exp. Med.* 162(4):1336-1349.

Nordoy, A. (1985). Dietary fatty acids, platelets, endothelial cells and coronary artery disease. *Acta Medica Scand.(Suppl).* 701:15.

Oconner, T. P., Roebuck, B. D., Campbell, T. C. (1985). Effect of dietary intake of fish oil and fish protein on the development of L-azaserine induced preneoplastic lesions in the rat pancreas. *J. Nat. Can. Inst.* 75(5):959-962.

Phillison, B. E. Rothrock, D. W. Connor, W. E. Harris, W. S., Illingworth, D. R. (1985). Reduction of plasma lipids, lipoproteins, and apoporteins by dietary fish oils in patients with hypertriglyceridemia. *N. Engl. J. Med.* 312(19):1210-1216.

Phillipson, B. E. Rothrock, D. W. Connor, W. E. Harris, W. S. Illingworth, D. R. (1985). Fish consumption and mortality from coronary heart disease. *New Eng. J. Med.* 313(13):824.

Podell, R. N. (1985). Nutritional treatment of rheumatoid arthritis. Can alterations in fat intake affect disease course? *Postgrad. Med.* 77(7):65-72.

Puustinen, T., et al. (1985). Fatty acid composition of 12 northern European fish species., *Acta Medica Scand.* 218(1):59-62.

Sanders, T. A. (1985). Influence of a fish-oil supplements on man. *Proc. Nutr. Soc.* 44(3):391-397.

Sanders, T. A. Sullivan, D. R. Reeve, J. Thompson, G. R. (1985). Triglyceride-lowering effect on marine polyunsaturates in patients with hypertriglyceridemia. *Arteriosclerosis* 5(5):459-465.

Shekelle, R. Paul, O. Syrock, A. Stamler, J. (1985). Fish consumption and mortality from coronary heart disease. *New Eng. J. Med.* 313(13):820.

Silberner, Joanne. (1985). Heart Disease, Let them eat fish. *Science News* May 11:295(1).

Simmons, L. A. Hickie, J. B. Balasubramaniam, S. (1985). On the effects of dietary N-3 fatty acids (maxEPA). on plasma lipids and lipoproteins in patients with hyperlipidaemia. *Atherosclerosis* 54(1):75-88.

Singer, P. Wirth, M. Berger., I. Voigt, S. Gerike, U. Godicke, W. Koberle, U. Heine, H. (1985). Influence on serum lipids, lipoproteins and blood pressure of mackerel and herring diet in patients with type IV and V hyperlipoproteinemia. *Atherosclerosis* 56(1):111-118.

Singer, P. Wirth, M. Godicke, W. Heine, H. (1985). Blood pressure lowering effect of eicosapentaenoic acid-rich diet in normotensive, hypertensive and hyperlipemic subjects. *Experientia* 41(4):462-454.

Skorepa, J. Hrabak, P. Zak, A. Zeman, M. Sindelkova, E. (1985). The effect of fish oils on plasma lipid levels in hyperlipidemics. *Cas. Lek. Cesk.* 124(31):970-973.

Terano, T., et al. (1985). Antiinflammatory effects of eicosapentaenoic acid, relevance to icosanoid formation., *Adv. Prostaglandin Thromboxane Leukotriene Res.* 15:253-255.

Tumura, Y. Hirai, A. Terano, T. Kumagai, A. Yoshida, S. (1985). Effects of eicosapentaenoic acid on hemostatic function and serum lipids in humans. *Adv. Prostaglandin Thromboxane Leukotriene Res.* 15:265-267.

Von Shackey, C., and Weber, P. (1985). Metabolism and effects on platelet function of the purified eicosapentaenoic and docosahexaenoic acids in humans. *J. Clin. Invest.* 76(5):2446-2450.

Von Shacky, C. Fischer, S. Weber, P. C. (1985). Long-term effects of dietary marine omega-3 fatty acids upon plasma and cellular lipids, platelet function, and eicosanoid formation in humans. *J. Clin. Invest.* 76(4):1626-1631.

Wallis, Claudia. (1985). Is seafood good for the heart? Eating some kinds of fish may reduce coronary disease. *Time* May 20:64(1).

Yamori, Y., et al. (1985). Comparison of serum phospholipid fatty acids among fishing and farming Japanese populations and American inlanders. *J. Nutr. Sci. Vitaminol.* 31(4):417-422.

No author. (1985). Reduction of plasma lipids and lipoproteins by marine fish oils. *Nutr. Rev.* 43(9):268-270.

No author. (1985). Healthy fats? (Fish oils). *Environment* April:22(1).

No author. (1985). Dietary fats and cancer., *Medical Hypothesis.* 17:351-362.

No author. (1935). Fish consumption and mortality from coronary artery disease. *New Eng J. Med.* 313:820.

No author. (1985). Blood pressure and lipid lowering effects of mackerel and herring diet in patients with mild essential hypertension. *Atherosclerosis* 56(2):223-235.

1984:

Ahmed, A. A. Houlb, B. J. (1984). Alteration and recovery of bleeding times, platelet aggregation and fatty acid composition of individual phospholipids in platelets of human subjects receiving a supplement of cod-liver oil. *Lipids* 19(8):617-624.

Bondi, A. Sklan, D. (1984). Vitamin A and carotene in animal nutrition. *Prog. Food Nutr. Sci.* 8(1-2):165-191.

Breniske, J. F., et al. (1984). Effects of therapy with cholestyramine on progression of coronary atherosclerosis, results of the NHLBI Type II coronary intervaention study. *Circulation.* 69(2):313-324.

Chesebro, J. Fuster, V. Elveback, L., et al. (1984). Effect of dipyridamole and aspirin on late vien graft patency after coronary bypass operations. *N. Engl. J. Med.* 310:209-214.

Clarke, S. D. (1984). Nutritional control of lipid synthesis. *ASDC. J. Dent. Child.* 51(3):218-221.

Driss, F. Vericel, E. Lagarde, M. Dechavanne, M. Darcet, P. (1984). Inhibition of platelet aggregation and thromboxane synthesis after intake of small amount of icosapentaenoic acid. *Thromb. Res.* 36(5):389-396.

Eichner, E. R. (1984). Platelets, carotids, and coronaries. Critique on antihrombotic role of antiplatelet agents, exercise, and certain diets. *Am. J. Med.* 77(3):513-523.

Fischer, S. Homigmann, G. Hora, C. Schimke, E. Beitz, J. Hanefeld, M. Leonhardt, W. Haller, H. Forster, W. Schliak, V. (1984). Results of linseed oil and olive oil therapy in hyperlipoproteinemia patients. *Dtsch. Z. Verdau. Stoffwechselkr.* 44(5):245-251.

Fischer, S., et al. (1984). Prostaglandin I3 is formed in vivo in man after dietary eicosapentaenoic acid. *Nature.* 307(5947):165-168.

Hamazaki, T. Nakazawa, R. Tateno, S. Shishido, H. Isoda, K. Hattori, Y. Yoshida, T. Fujita, T. Yano, S. Kumagai, A. (1984). Effects of fish oil rich in eicosapentaenoic acid on serum lipid in hyperlipdemic hemodialysis patients. *Kidney Int.* 26(1):81-84.

Harris, W. S. Connor, W. E. Inkeles, S. B. Illingworth, D. R. (1984). Dietary omega-3 fatty acids prevent carbohydrate-induced hypertriglyceridemia. *Metabolism* 33(11):1016-1019.

Harris, W. S. Conno, W. E. Lindsey, S. (1984). Will dietary omega-3 fatty acids change the composition of human milk? *Am. J. Clin. Nutr.* 40(4):780-785.

Illingsworth, D. R. Harris, W. S. Connor, W. E. (1984). Inhibition of low density lipoprotein synthesis by dietary omega-3 fatty acids in humans. *Arteriosclerosis* 4(3):270-275.

Kromhout, D., and Coulander C. D. L. (1984). Diet, prevalence and 10-year mortality from coronary heart disease in 871 middle-aged men. The Zutphen study. *Am. J. Epidem.* 119:733-741.

McGree D. L., et al. (1984). Ten-year incidence of coronary heart disease in the Honolulu Heart Program, Relationship to nutrient intake. *Am. J. Epidemiol.* 119:667-676.

Moncada, S. Vane, J. R. (1984). Prostacyclin and its clinical applications. *Ann. Clin. Res.* 16(5-6):241-252.

Nestel, P. J. Connor, W. E. Reardon, M. F. Connor, S. Wong, S. (1984). Boston, R. Suppression by diets rich in fish oil of very low density lipoprotein production in man. *J. Clin. Invest.* 74(1):82-89.

Nordy, A. Lagarde, M. Renaud, S. (1984) Platelets during alimentary hyper-lipaemia induced by cream and cod liver oil. *Eur. J. Clin. Invest* 14(5):339-345.

Otsuji, S., Kamada, T., Yamashita, T., Soejima, Y., Setoyama, S., Hashiguchi, J., Chuman, Y. (1984). The influence of dietary sardine oil (eicosapentaenoic acid). on the erythrocyte membrane fluidity in diabetic patients. *Rinsho-Byori* 32(7):764-761.

Podell, R. N. (1984). The "Tomato Effect" in clinical nutrition. New treatments languishing on the vine? *Postgrad. Med.* 76(8):49-52, 61-63, 65.

Popp, Snijbers C. Schouten, J. A. De Jong, A. P. Van Der Veen, E. A. (1984). Effect of dietary cod-liver oil on the lipid composition of human erythrocyte membranes. *Scand. J. Clin. Lab. Invest.* 44(1):39-46.

Prescott, S. M. (1984). The effect of EPA on leukotriene B production by human neutrophils. *J. Biol. Chem.* 259(12):7615-7621.

Rylance, P. B. George, M. P. Saynor, R. Weston, M. J. (1984). A pilot study of the use of MaxEPA in haemodialysis patients. *Br. J. Clin. Pract.* 31:49-54.

Saynor, R. Verel, D. Gillott, T. (1984). The effect of MaxEPA on the serum lipids, platelets, bleeding time and GTN consumption. *Br. J. Clin. Pract.* 31:70-74.

Saynor, R. (1984). Effects of omega-3 fatty acids on serum lipids [Letter]. *Lancet* 2(8404):696-697.

Saynor, R. Verel, D. G llott, T. (1984). The long-term effect of dietary supplemen-tation with fish lipid concentrate on serum lipids, bleeding time, platelets and angina. *Atherosclerosis* 50(1):3-10.

Schimke, E., Hildebrandt, R., Beitz, J., Schimke, I., Semmler, S. Homigmann, G., Mest, H. J., Schliack, V. (1984). Influence of a cod liver diet in diabetics Type I on fatty acid patterns and platelet aggregation. *Biomed-Biochem Acta* 43(8-9):S351-S353.

Singer, P. Honigmann, G. Schliack, V. (1984). Negative correlation of eicosapentaenoicacid and lipid accumluation in hepatocytes of diabetics. *Biomed. Biochim. Acta.* 43(8-9):S438-442.

Singer, P. Wirth, M. Voigt, S. Zimontkowski, S. Godicke, W. Heine, H. (1984). Clinical studies on lipid and blood pressure lowering effect of eicosapentaenoic acid-rich diet. *Biomed. Biochim. Acta.* 43(8-9):S421-425.

Walsh, G. P. (1984). A GP's use of omega-3 lipids in coronary heart disease. *Br. J. Clin. Pract.* 31:75-76.

Woodcock, B. E. Smith, E. Lambert, W. H. Jones, W. M. Galloway, J. H. Greaves, M. Preston, F. E. (1984). Beneficial effect of fish oil on blood viscosity in peripheral vascular disease. *Br. Med. J. (Clin. Res.).* 288(6417):592-594.

Vaughn, Lewis. (1984). The fish oil factor, Healthy heart gift from the sea. *Prevention* March:64(6).

No author. (1984). Eat your fish oil, dear (new treatment for cardiovascular disease). *Environment* May:24(1).

No author. (1984). Negative correlation of EPA and lipid accumulation in hepatocytes of diabetics. *Biomed. Biochem. Acta.* 43(8-9):99-108.

No author. (1984). National Institute of Health Consensus Conference on the Treatment of Hypertriglyceridemia, *J.A.M.A.* 251:1196-1200.

No author. (1984). Lipids Research Clinics Coronary Prevention Trial Results, II. The relationship of reduction in incidence of coronary heart disease to cholesterol lowering. *J.A.M.A.* 24:365.

No author. (1984). Lipids Research Clinics Coronary Primary Prevention Trial Results, I. Reduction in incidence of coronary heart disease. *J.A.M.A.* 241:351.

1983:

Bradlow, B. A. Chetty, N. Van Der Westhuyzen, J. Mendelsohn, D. Gibson, J. E. (1983). The effects of a mixed fish diet on platelet function, fatty acids and serum lipids. *Thromb. Res.* 29(6):561-568.

Brox J. H., et al. (1983). Effect of cod liver oil on platelets and coagulation in familial hypercholesterolemia. *Acta Medica Scand.* 213:137-144

Brox, J. H. Killie, J.E. Osterud, B. Holme, S. Nordy, S. (1983). Effects of cod liver oil on platelets and coagulation in familial hypercholesterolemia (type IIA). *Acta. Med. Scand.* 213(2):137-144.

Brox, J. H., et al. (1983). The effect of polyunsaturated fatty acids on endothelial cells and their production of prostacyclin, thromboxane and platelet inhibitory activity. *Thromb. Heamost.* 50(4):762-767.

Enhorn, D. L. H., et al. (1983). Eskimos and their diets. *Lancet* 1:1335.

Fehily, A. M. Burr, M. L. Phillips, K. M. Deadman, N. M.(1983). The effect of fatty fish on plasma lipid and lipoprotein concentrations. *Am. J. Clin. Nutr.* 38(3):349-351

Fredericks, Carlton. (1983). There's more in fish than vitamins A and D. (Eicosapentaenoic acid combats multiple sclerosis). (Column). *Prevention* August:130(2).

Fredericks, Carlton. (1983). More fish, less heart disease? (Fish oil inhibits blood platelet clumping). (Column). *Prevention* May:31(2)

Fredericks, Carlton. (1983). A fish story may be true, Seafood versus heart disease. (Fish oils). (Column). *Prevention* March:30(1).

Harris. W. Connor, w. McMurray, M. (1983). The comparative reductions of the plasma lipid an lipoporteins of dietary polyunsaturated fats, Salmon oil versus vegetable oils. *Metabolism* 32:179-184.

Jorgensen, K. A. Dyerberg, J. (1983). Platelets and atherosclerosis. *Adv. Nutr. Res.* 5:57-75.

Kawamura, M. Naito, C. Hayashi, H. Hashimoto, Y. Kato, H. Matsushima, T. (1983). Effects of 4 weeks' intake of polyunsaturated fatty acid ethylester rich in eicosapentaenoic acid (ethylester). on plasma lipids, plasma and platelet phospholipid fatty acid composition and platelet aggregation, A double blind study *Nippon Naika Gakkai Zasshi* 72(1):18-24.

Lorenz, R. Spengler, U. Gischer, S., et. al. (1983). Platelet function, thromboxane formation and blood pressure control during supplementation of Western diet with cod liver oil. *Circulation* 67:504-511.

Miettinen, T. A. Althan, G. Huttunen, J. K. Pikkarainen, J. Naukkarian, V., Mattilla, S. Kumlin, T. (1983). Serum selenium concentration related to myocardial infarction and fatty acid content of serum lipids. *Br. Med. J. (Clin Res).* 287(6391):517-519.

Moncada, S. (1983). Biology and therapeutic potential of prostacyclin. *Stroke* 14(2):157-168.

Morita, I. Takahisni, R. Ito, H. Orimo, H. Murota, S. (1983). Increases arachidonic acid content in platelet phospholipids from diabetic patients. *Prostaglandins Leukotrienes Med.* 11(1):33-41.

Mortensen, J. Z. Schmidt, E. B. Nielsen, A. H. Dyerberg, J. (1983). The effect of N-6 and N-3 polyunsaturated fatty acids on hemostasis, blood lipids and blood pressure. *Thromb. Haemost.* 50(2):543-546.

Nagakawa, N. Orimc, H. Harasawa, M. Morita, I. Yashiro, K. Murota, S. (1983). Effect of eicosapentaenoic acid on the platelet aggregation and composition of fatty acid in man. A double blind study. *Atherosclerosis* 47(1):71-75.

Pitt, B. E., et al. (1983). Prostaglandins and prostaglandin inhibitors in ischemic heart disease. *Ann. Int. Med.* 99:83.

Rylance, P. B. George, M. P. Saynor, R., et al. (1983). A pilot study of the use of MaxEPA in haemodialysis patients. *Br. J. Med.* Suppl 31:49-51.

Sanders, T. A. Hochland, M. C. (1983). A comparison of the influence on plasma lipids and platelets function of supplements of omega 3 and omega 6 polyunsaturated fatty acids. *Br. J. Nutr.* 50(3):521-529.

Sanders, T. A. Roshanai, F. (1983). The influence of different types of omega 3 polyunsaturated fatty acids on blood lipids and platelet function in healthy volunteers. *Clin. Sci.* 64(1):91-99.

Sanders, T. A. (1983). Dietary fat and platelet function. *Clin. Sci.* 65(4):343-350.

Saynor, R. Verel, D. (1983). Eskimos and their diets [Letter]. *Lancet* 1(8337):1335.

Singer, P. Jaeger, W. Wirth, M. Voigt, S. Naumann, E. Zimotkowski, S. Hajdu, I. Goedicke, W. (1983). Lipid and blood pressure-lowering effect of mackerel diet in man. *Atherosclerosis* 49(1):99-108.

Terano, T. Hirai, A. Hamazaki, T. Kobayashi, S. Fujita, T. Tamura, Y. Kumagai, A. (1983). Effect of oral administration of highly purified eicosapentaenoic acid on platelet function blood viscosity and red cell deformability in healthy human subjects. *Atherosclerosis* 46(3):312-332.

Thorngren, M., et al. (1983). Effects of acetylsalicylic acid on platelet aggregation before and during increase in dietary EPA. *Haemostasis* 13(4):244-247.

Thorngren, M. Gustafson, A. (1983). Effects of acetylsalicylic acid and dietary intervention on primary hemostasis. *Am. J. Med.* (Suppl):66-69.

Tremoli,E. Galli, C. Socini, A. Paoletti, R. (1983). Postaglandins in the cardiovascular system, Dietary lipid modulation. *Prev. Med.* 12(1):11-15.

No author. (1983). Eskimo diets and diseases. *Lancet* ii:1139-1141.

No author. (1983). Comparative reductions of the plasma lipids and lipoproteins by dietary polyunsaturated fats: salmon oil vs. vegetable oil. *Metabolism* 32:279-184.

1982:

Ackman, R. G. (1982). Fatty acid composition of fish oils. in "Nutritional Evaluation of Long-chain Fatty Acids in Fish Oils" (S. M. Barlow and M. E. Stansby, eds.)., Academic Press, pp. 25-88. New York.

Bechtel, Stefan. (1982). Fish oil, new harpoon against heart disease. (Lowers blood fats). *Prevention* December:73(4).

Connor, W. E., (1982). Polyunsaturated fatty acids, hyperlipidemia, and thrombosis. *Arteriosclerosis* 2:87-113.

Cordova, C. Nusca, A. Violi, F. Perrone, A. De Mattia, G. Alessandri, C. Salvadori, F. (1982). Effects of cod liver oil on platelet aggergation and lipid parameters. *Clin. Ther.* 102(3):277-281.

Dyerberg, J. Bang, H. O. (1982). A hypothesis on the development of acute myocardial infarction in Greenlanders. *Scand. J. Clin. Lab. Invest.* [Suppl] 16:17-13.

Dyerberg, J. Jergensen, K. A. (1982). Marine oils and thrombogenesis. *Prog. Lipid. Res.* 21(4):255-269.

Felman, Bruce. (1982). Linoleic acid–A fat you can't live without. (safflower, sunflower, corn oils, et al.). *Prevention* April:71(4).

Goodnight, S. H., JR. Harris, W. S. Connor, W. E. Illingsworth, D. R. (1982). Polyunsaturated fatty acids, hyperlipidemia, and thrombosis. *Arteriosclerosis* 2(2):87-113,

Haagsma, N. C., van Gent, C. M., Luten, J. B., deJong R. W., and van Doorn, E. (1982). Preparation of omega-3 fatty acid concentrate from cod liver oil. *J. Am. Oil Chem. Soc.* 59:117-118.

Harris, W. S., et al. (1982). Dietary fish oils, plasmalipids and platelets in man. *Prog. Lip. Res.* 20:75-79.

Hay, C. R. Durber, A. P. Saynor, R. (1982). Effect of fish oil on platelet kinetics in patients with ischaemic heart disease. *Lancet* 1(8284):1269-1270.

Hirai, A. Terano, T. Hamazaki, T. Sajiki, J. Kondo, S. Ozawa, A. Fujita, T. Miyamota, T. Tamura, Y. Kumagai, A. (1982). The effects of the oral administratin of fish oil concentrate on the release and the metabolism of C[14] arachidnoic acid and C[14] eicosapentaenoic acid by human platelets. *Thromb. Res.* 28(3):285-298.

Johnson, G. Timothy. (1982). Health, fish oil & heart disease; *Washington Post* October 3:17.

Kagawa, Y. Nishizawa, M. Suzuki, M. Miyatake, T. Hamanoto, T. Goto, K. Motonaga, E. Izumikawa, H. Hirata, H. Ebihara, A. (1982). Eicosapolyenoic acids of serum lipids of Japanese islanders with low incidence of cardiovascular diseases. *J. Nutri. Sci. Vitaminol (Tokyo).* 28(4):441-453.

Lea, E. J. Jones, S. P. Hamilton, D. V. (1982). The fatty acids of erythrocytes in myocardial infarction patients. *Atherosclerosis* 41(2-3):363-369.

Lockette, W. E., Webb, R. C., Culp, B. R., and Pitt, B. (1982). Vascular reactivity and high dietary eicosapentaenoic acid. *Prostaglandins* 24:631-639.

Needleman, P. E., et al. (1982). Fatty acids as sources of potential magic bullets for modification of platelet and vascular function. *Prog. Lip. Res.* 20:415-422.

Miettinen, T. A. Naukkarinen, V. Huttunen, J. K. Mattilla, S. Kumlin, T. (1982). Fatty acid composition of serum lipids predicts myocardial infarction. *Br. Med. J. (Clin Res)*. 285(6347):993-996.

Okabe, H. Kanai, A. Noma, A. (1982). Effect of aging on the concentrations of arachidonic acid and eicosapentaeonic acid in human serum lipids. *Nippon Romen Gakkai Zasshi* 19(3):279-284.

Saynor, R. Verel, D. (1982). Eicosapentaenoic acid, bleeding time, and serum lipids [Letter]. *Lancet* 2(8292):272.

Talesnik, J., and Hsia, J. C. (1982). Coronary flow reactions to arachidonic acid are inhibited by docosahexaenoic acid. *J. Pharm.* 80:255-258.

Vas Dias, F. W., et al. (1982). The effect of polyunsaturated fatty acids of the n-3 and n-6 series of platelet aggregation and platelet and aortic fatty acid composition in rabbits. *Atherosclerosis* 43:245-257.

No author. (1982). The fish oil factor: Why do eskimos have so few heart attacks? *Health* April:30(1).

No author. (1981). Fish oil for prevention of Atherosclerosis. *Med. Lett. Drugs Ther.* 24(622):99-100.

1981

Budowski, P. (1981). Review:Nutritional effects of w-3 polyunsaturated fatty acids. *Isr. J. Med. Sci.* 17:223-231.

Brox, J. H. Killie, J. E. Gunnes, S. Nordy, A. (1981). The effect of cod liver oil and corn oil on platelets and vessel wall in man. *Thromb. Haemost.* 46(3):604-611.

Bronsgeest, S., et al. (1981). The effect of various intakes of w-3 fatty acids on the blood lipid composition in healthy human subjects. *Am. J. Clin. Nutr.* 34:1752-1757.

Bronsgeest-Schoute, H. C. Ruiter, A. (1981). Specific effect of highly unsaturated lipids of animal origin on the blood lipid composition (Author's transl). *Tijdschr Diergeneeskd* 106(5):257-264.

Dyerberg, J. (1981). Platelet-Vessel wall interaction, influence of diet. *Philos. Trans. R. Soc. Lond. [Biol]* 294(1072):373-381.

Goodnight, S. H., Jr. Harris, W. S. Connor, W. E. (1981). The effects of dietary omega 3 fatty acids on platelet composition and function in man, A prospective, controlled study. *Blood* 58(5):880-885.

Katan, M. B., and Beynen, A. C. (1981). Linoleic acid consumption and coronary heart disease in USA and U.K, *Lancet* 2:371.

Kobayashi, S., et al. (1981). Reduction of blood viscosity by eicosapentaenoic acid. Lancet 2:197.

Murphy, R. C. Pickett, W. C. Culp, B. R. Lands, W. E. (1981). Tetraene and pentaene leukaktrienes, selective production from murine mastocytoma cells after dietary manipulation. Prostaglandins 22(4):613-622.

Sanders, T. A. Vickers, M. Haines, A. P. (1981). Effect of blood lipids and haemostasis of supplement of cod-liver oil, rich in eicosapentaenoic and docosahexaenoic acids, in healthy young men. Clin. Sci. 61(3):317-324.

Shekelle, R. B., et al. (1981). Diet, serum cholesterol, and death from coronary heart disease, The Western Electric study. New Eng. J. Med. 304:65-70.

Singer, P. Honigmann, G. Schliack, V. (1981). Fatty acid composition of triglycerides in inflammatory liver diseases in diabetics with and without hyperlipoporteiremia. Z. Gesamte. Inn. Med. 36(15):513-519.

Thorngren, M. Gustafson, A. (1981). Effects of 11 week increases in dietary eicosapentaencic acid on bleeding time, lipids, and platelet aggregation. Lancet 2(8257):1190-1193.

No author. (1981). Experimental myocardial infarction and fish oil. Nutr. Rev. 39(8):316-317.

No Author. (1981). Diet and its relation to coronary heart disease and death in three populations. Circulation 63:500-515.

No Author. (1981). Fish oil feeding lowers thromboxane and prostacyclin production by rat platelets and aorta and does not result in the formation of prostaglandin I. Prostaglandins 21:727-738.

1980:

Bang, H. O., and Dyberg, J. (1980). The bleeding tendency in Greenland Eskimos. Dan. Med Bull. 27:202-205.

Bang, H. O. Dyerberg, J. Sinclair, H. M. (1980). The composition of the eskimo food in northwestern Greenland. Am. J. Clin. Nutr. 33(12):2657-2661.

Cohen, I. (1980). Platelet structure and function role of prostaglandins. Ann. Clin. Lab. Sci. 0(3):187-194.

Gudbjarnason, S. (1980)). Pathophysiology of long-chain polyene fatty acids in heart muscle. Nutr. Metab. 24 Suppl 1:142-146.

Hirai, A. Hamazaki, T. Terano, T. Nishikawa, T. Tamura, T. Kumagai, A. Sajaki, J. (1980). Eicosapentaenoic acid and platelet function in Japanese. Lancet 2:1132-1133.

Hooper, Judith. (1980). Fish oil. Omni September:42(1).

Hornstra, G. (1980). Dietary prevention of coronary heart disease. Effect of dietary fats on arterial thrombosis. Postgrad. Med. J. 56(658):563-570.

Kromann, N., and Green, A. (1980). Epidemiological studies in the Upernavik district, Greenland. *Acta Med. Scand.* 208:401-406.

Lands, W. E. Pitt, B. W. Culp, B. R. (1980). Recent concepts on platelet function and dietary lipids in coronary thrombosis, vasospasm and angina. *HERZ* 5(1):34-41.

Pitcairn, Richard H. (1980). Cod-liver oil to the rescue, A case of corneal ulcer. (Your healthy pet). *Prevention* September:148(4).

Seiss, W., et al. (1980). Platelet membrane fatty acids, platelet aggregation and thromboxane formation during a mackerel diet. *Lancet* 1:441-444.

Srivastava, K. C. (1980). Effects of dietary fatty acids, prostaglandins and related compounds on the role of platelets in thrombosis. *Biochem. Exp. Biol.* 16(3):317-338.

Singer, P. Honigmann, G. Schliack, V. (1980). Decrease of eicosapentaenoic acid in fatty liver of diabetic subjects. *Prostaglandins Med.* 5(3):183-200.

Uhlaner, Jonathan. (1980). Let your heart off the hook with fish. *Prevention* August:52(4).

No author. (1980). Lipids, platelets, and atherosclerosis. *Lancet* 1(8166):464-465.

No author. (1980). Fish-oil diet. *Science Digest* November-December:108(1).

No author. (1980). The effect of dietary supplementation of fish oil on experimental myocardial infarction. *Prostaglandins* 31:1021-1031.

1979:

Culp, B. R., et al. (1979). Inhibition of prostaglandins synthesis by eicosapentaenoic acid. *Prostaglandin Med.* 3:269.

Dyerberg J. Bang, H. O. (1979). Haeomostatic function and platelet polyunsaturated fatty acids in Eskimos. *Lancet* 2:433-455.

Taylor, T. G., Gibney, M. J., and Morgan, J. B. (1979). Haemostatic function and polyunsaturated fatty acids. *Lancet* 2:1378.

No author. (1979). Fish, a healthy food dictionary. *Prevention* November:193(3).

No author. (1979). Cod-liver oil for your body machinery. *Prevention* March:68(4).

No author. (1979). Fish oil and heart disease. *New York Times* December 17:16.

1978:

Angelico, F. Amodeo, P. (1978). Eicosapentaenoic acid and prevention of atherosclerosis [Letter]. *Lancet* 2(8088):531.

Burn, J. H. (1978). Early observations and their importance today. I. Diabetes in childhood, II. Theophylline in myasthenia gravis III. properties of cod liver oil. *J. Pharm. Pharmacol.* 30(12):779-782.

Dyerberg, J Bang, H. O. Stofferson, E. Moncada, S. Vane, J. R. (1978). Eicosapentaenoic acid prevention of thrombosis and atherosclerosis? *Lancet* 2(8081):117-119.

Ruiter, A., et al (1978). The influence of dietary mackerel oil on the condition of organs and on blood lipid composition on the young growing pig. *Am. J. Clin. Nutr.* 31:2159-2166.

Stansby, M E. (1978). Development of fish oil industry in the United States. *J. Am. Oil Chem. Soc.* 55:238-243

Von Lossonczy, T O. Buiter, A. Bornsgeest-Schoute, H. C (1978). The effect of a fish diet on serum lipids in healthy human subjects. *Am. J. Clin. Nutr.* 31:1340-1346.

No author. (978). EPA and prevention of thrombosis and atherosclerosis. *Lancet* 2:117-119.

Kachorovski, B. V. Zhoglo, F. A. Zaverbnyi, M. I. (1977). Total lipid content in the blood after using fish oil in natural and emulsified forms. *Farmatsia* 26(5):86.

Robertson, T., et al. (1977). Epidemiologic studies of coronary disease and stroke in Japanese men living in Japan, Hawaii and California. *Am. J. Cardiol.* 39:244

Singer, P. Gnauck, G. Honigmann, G. Schliack, V. Laeuter, J. (1977). The fatty acid composition of triglycerides in arteries, depot fat and serum of amputated diabetics. *Atherosclerosis* 28(1):87-92

No author. (1977). Plasma cholesterol concentration in caucasian Danes and green-land Eskimos. *Am. J. Clin. Nutr* 28:958-966.

1976:

Bang, H. O. Dyerberg, J. Hjorne, N. (1976). Fatty acid composition of food consumed by Greenland Eskimos. *Acta. Med. Scand.* 200:69-73.

1975:

Dyerberg, J Bang, H. O. Hjorne, N. (1975). The composition of the plasma lipids in Greenland Eskimos. *Am. J. Clin. Nutr.* 28:958.

1972:

Connor, W. E., and Conner, S. I. (1972). The key role of nutritional factors in the prevention of coronary heart disease. *Prev. Med* 1:49.

Feldman, S. A., et al. (1972). Lipid and cholesterol metabolism in Alaskan Arctic Eskimos. *A. M. A. Arch. Pathol.* 94:42-58.

Nelson, A. M. (1972). Diet therapy in coronary disease-effect on mortality of high-protein, high-seafood, fat-controlled diet. *Geriatrics* 27:103.

1971:

Bang, H.O., Dyberg, J., Nielsen, A. B. (1971). Plasma lipid and lipoprotein pattern in greenland west-coast Eskimos. *Lancet.* 1(7701):1143-1146.

Kannel, W. B. (1971). Serum cholesterol, lipoproteins, and the risk of coronary heart disease: The Framingham study. *Am. Int. Med.* 74:1-11.

Kiefer, R. R., et al. (1971). Effect of dietary fish oil on the fatty acid composition and palatability of pig tissues. *Fishery Bulletin* 69:281-302.

1970:

Arthaud, B. (1970). Cause of death in 339 alaskan natives as detrmined by autopsy. *A. M. A. Archives Path.* 90:433-438.

Keys, A. (1970). Coronary heart disease in seven countries. *Circulation* 41(S):1-211.

1969:

Kifer, R. R., and Miller D. (1969). Fish oils-fatty acid composition energy values, metabolism, and vitamin content. *Fish Ind.* 5:25.

1967:

Kakuk, T. J. Olson, C. (1967). Dietary influence of a cod liver oil fraction on avian lymphocytoma. *Avian Dis* 11(3):336-341.

1962:

Pfeifer, J. J., Janssen, F., Muesing, R., and Lundberg, W. O. (1972). The lipid depressant activities of whole fish and their component oils. *J. Am. Chem. Soc.* 39:292-296.

1960:

Gottman, A. W., et al. (1960). A report of 103 autopsies on alaskan natives, *A.M.A. Arch. Patho.* 70:117-124.

1959:

No author. (1959). Cholesterol-lowering oils. *Science News Letter* September 24:271.

1953:

Enos, W. F., et al. (1953). Coronary disease among U.S. soldiers killed in action in Korea. *J.A.M.A.* 152:1090-1093.

Sinclair, H. M. (1953). The diet of Canadian Indians and Eskimos. *Proc. Nutr. Soc.* 12-69-82.

1952:

Brown, M., et al. (1952). The occurence of cancer in an Eskimo. *Cancer* 5:142-143.

1950:

Wilber, C. G., and Levine, V. E. (1959). Fat metabolism in Alaskan Eskimos. *Exp. Med. Surg.* 8:422-425.

1937:

Corcoran, A. C., and Rabinowitch, I. M. (1937). A study of the blood lipids and blood protein in Canadian Eastern Arctic Eskimos. *Biochem J.* 31:543-548.

1914:

Krogh, A., and Krogh, M. A study of the diet and metabolism of Eskimos undertaken in 1908 on an expedition to Greenland. *Medd Greenland* 51(1):1-2.

19

INDEX